BRIEF THERAPY FOR POST-TRAUMATIC STRESS DISORDER

DURHAM

WILEY SERIES
in
BRIEF THERAPY AND COUNSELLING

Editor

Windy Dryden

BRIEF THERAPY FOR POST-TRAUMATIC STRESS DISORDER

Traumatic incident reduction and related techniques

Stephen Bisbey
The Bisbeys Partnership and Research/Clinician, London Transport Trauma Research and Counselling Unit

and

Lori Beth Bisbey
The Bisbeys Partnership and Senior Research/Clinician, London Transport Trauma Research and Counselling Unit

JOHN WILEY & SONS

Chichester · New York · Weinheim · Brisbane · Singapore · Toronto

National   01243 779777
International (+44) 1243 779777
e-mail (for orders and customer service enquiries): cs-books@wiley.co.uk
Visit our Home Page on http://www.wiley.co.uk
or http://www.wiley.com

Reprinted April 1999

Other Wiley Editorial Offices

John Wiley & Sons, Inc., 605 Third Avenue,
New York, NY 10158-0012, USA

Wiley-VCH Verlag GmbH, Pappelallee 3, D-69469
Weinheim, Germany

Jacaranda Wiley Ltd, 33 Park Road, Milton,
Queensland 4064, Australia

John Wiley & Sons (Asia) Pte Ltd, 2 Clementi Loop #02-01,
Jin Xing Distripark, Singapore 129809

John Wiley & Sons (Canada) Ltd, 22 Worcester Road,
Rexdale, Ontario M9W 1L1, Canada

Library of Congress Cataloging-in-Publication Data

Bisbey, Stephen.
    Brief therapy for post-traumatic stress disorder : traumatic
incident reduction and related techniques / Stephen Bisbey and Lori
Beth Bisbey.
        p.   cm. — (Wiley series in brief therapy and counselling)
    Includes bibliographical references and index.
    ISBN 0–471–975672 (paper)
    1. Post-traumatic stress disorder—Treatment. 2. Brief
psychotherapy. I. Bisbey, Lori Beth. II. Title. III. Series.
RC552.P67B575 1998
616.85´21—dc21   97–45185
                                                                   CIP

British Library Cataloguing in Publication Data

A catalogue record for this book is available from the British Library

ISBN 0-471-97567-2

Typeset in 10/12pt Palatino from the author's disks by Dorwyn Ltd, Rowlands Castle, Hants
Printed and bound in Great Britain by Biddles Ltd, Guildford and King's Lynn.
This book is printed on acid-free paper responsibly manufactured from sustainable forestry, for which as least two trees are planted for each one used for paper production.

CONTENTS

To our Families
Especially Stephen's Father, Jack Bisbey
and
Lori's Mom, Dad and Grandma

ABOUT THE AUTHORS

Stephen Bisbey has been in private counselling practice for the past 15 years. He specializes in trauma (treatment, training, research and supervision), relationship difficulties and couples work, and the treatment of cult survivors. He has been involved in media work relating to all of these areas.

Mr Bisbey is a Certified Trauma Specialist and works at Victim Support Lambeth weekly seeing traumatized victims of crime. He is a research clinician at the London Transport Trauma Research and Counselling Centre where he is working on a large treatment outcome research project. He spends the rest of his working time seeing clients in private practice, supervising mental health professionals working with traumatized clients, and designing treatment techniques and training programmes relating to his speciality areas.

Mr Bisbey has designed training materials for the staff support scheme of the East Anglian Ambulance NHS Trust, the 'buddy scheme' for London Transport. He is co-author of a variety of training manuals including *Advanced Traumatic Incident Reduction* and author of a variety of articles on structured person-focused counselling techniques. Mr Bisbey has presented at conferences in the UK, the USA and Europe on trauma and has been co-organizer of four conferences for trauma practitioners in the UK.

Lori Beth Bisbey received her MA and PhD in clinical psychology from California School of Professional Psychology, San Diego. She has been involved in clinical work for the past ten years, having spend the past six years in private practice with Stephen Bisbey. She specializes in trauma (recognition, treatment, research, supervision and training), psycho-diagnostics and forensic work. Her experience includes work in the US federal prison service, considerable work preparing medico-legal reports in civil, criminal and family matters in the USA, the UK and Ireland.

Since 1995, Dr Bisbey has been the external consultant for the staff support scheme of the East Anglian Ambulance NHS Trust. She divides the rest of her time between London Transport where she heads a treatment outcome research project, Victim Support Lambeth where she supervises a practicum for social work, counselling and psychology students involving trauma counselling, and private practice where she provides treatment for traumatized clients (particularly clients with dual diagnoses), supervises mental health professionals and does forensic/medico-legal work.

Dr Bisbey regularly provides training for mental health professionals on a variety of subjects. She has co-authored a variety of treatment manuals including the *Advanced Traumatic Incident Reduction* workshop. She has done media work relating to her speciality areas. Dr Bisbey has presented at conferences in the UK, the USA and Europe on trauma and has been co-organizer of four conferences for trauma practitioners in the UK.

SERIES PREFACE

In recent years, the field of counselling and psychotherapy has become preoccupied with brief forms of intervention. While some of this interest has been motivated by expediency – reducing the amount of help that is offered to clients to make the best use of diminishing resources – there has also developed the view that brief therapy may be the treatment of choice for many people seeking therapeutic help. It is with the latter view in mind that the Wiley Series in Brief Therapy and Counselling was developed.

This series of practical texts considers different forms of brief therapy and counselling as they are practised in different settings and with different client groups. While no book can substitute for vigorous training and supervision, the purpose of the books in the present series is to provide clear guides for the practice of brief therapy and counselling, which is here defined as lasting 25 sessions or less.

Windy Dryden
Series Editor

PREFACE

We were very pleased to be asked by Professor Dryden to contribute to this Brief Therapy and Counselling series. We have long felt that Post-Traumatic Stress Disorder is best treated in a brief therapy framework. Post-Traumatic Stress Disorder and trauma in general have become more and more recognized in the United Kingdom over the past ten years. More counsellors are being presented with traumatized clients and it is our hope that this book will assist them to choose and utilize appropriate and effective brief therapy methods to work with these clients. We hope that we have highlighted the differences between approaching trauma using a trauma-specific model which incorporates a holistic context and approaching trauma from a more traditional framework.

We would like to take this opportunity to thank a variety of people who have helped and supported us during this endeavour. We thank all our colleagues who were understanding when we became too distracted to complete some of our correspondence in a timely manner. We thank all the students who have attended Traumatic Incident Reduction and Advanced Traumatic Incident Reduction workshops. Their comments and suggestions were very helpful to us in the writing of this book. We thank all the people we have supervised in this field for their comments, suggestions and problems which have encouraged us to think and revise our models and our applications. Most of all, we thank our clients whose courage and persistence in the face of overwhelming trauma continues to touch us on such a deep level.

We thank our families and friends – too many to mention by name – for their unerring love and support as well as understanding when we had less time than we would have liked to spend with them.

We thank the publishing staff at John Wiley & Sons for being patient with us and for their help in preparing the manuscript for publication.

A few people deserve specific thanks by name: Dr G. Robert Baker, whose role of 'devil's advocate' in discussions over the years has enhanced our understanding and helped us clarify the stance we have taken in treating Post-Traumatic Stress Disorder; Clay Foreman for discussions that helped us to clarify where our stance placed us in the field; Gerald French for being so 'unbelievably cool' and offering friendship, encouragement, dynamic debate and the first TIR workshop manual which provided fertile ground for innovation; Dr Frank Gerbode for developing TIR, providing many hours of stimulating discussion and debate on technical and philosophical issues, for offering friendship, support and encouragement and for being so gracious when we started tinkering with his method; and the technical symposium group whose support, knowledge and feedback are much appreciated. In addition, we thank our editor, Professor Windy Dryden, for his patience, encouragement and direct editing style which we believe improved the final manuscript.

We give extra special thanks to the clients who have allowed their session material (and therefore their lives) to be disclosed in this book. They have all expressed the wish that counsellors would learn from their experiences. We could not have completed this project without their contributions and we are forever grateful.

ACKNOWLEDGEMENTS

We would like to thank again Gerald French for his kind permission to adapt and reprint material from the TIR Workshop manual and Dr Frank Gerbode for his kind permission to adapt and reprint material from his book, his TIR course manual and the TIR Workshop manual.

Our thanks to the American Psychiatric Association for permission to reprint the diagnoses for Acute Stress Disorder and Post-Traumatic Stress Disorder from the *Diagnostic and Statistical Manual of Mental Disorders – IV*.

HOW TO USE THIS BOOK

This book is designed to be used by counsellors **in conjunction with specific training in Traumatic Incident Reduction** and is **not** intended as a substitute for actual training. Though the model and the applications from the model seem simple, there is considerable skill involved in using these applications properly. Training workshops are usually four to five days in length and a large portion of the workshop is experiential practice of each of the techniques taught. This supervised practice is essential and without it counsellors may find the applications to be ineffective or could even further traumatize the client. This book can be profitably used as an adjunct to a training manual.

Gerbode (1989) intended TIR as a technique that can be used by trained counsellors as well as by people involved in self-help and peer-support work. We have some very definite biases on the efficacy of the technique without the appropriate training and/or without the practitioner having a background and experience in counselling. Our views differ somewhat from those of French and Gerbode (1995) and are outlined here.

The standard basic workshop, as we administer it in the UK, runs for five days and covers the areas outlined in this book. At the end of the workshop, we expect that the majority of experienced counsellors will feel some degree of confidence in using these techniques with appropriate clients with minimal supervision.* Free supervision (within reason) via telephone, fax or e-mail is provided for three months following the workshops we teach.

---

* Our definition of minimal supervision: Supervision that happens less than once weekly – where a counsellor seeks help on difficult clients only. Regular supervision happens at least once weekly and the counsellor presents the progress of a variety of his cases – regularly submitting audio tapes and session transcripts for comments from the supervisor. Peer supervision is when counsellors discuss cases with each other in a less formal manner. We believe counsellors should be involved in at least peer supervision on a regular basis (e.g. weekly).

With complex sessions, a supervisor can often provide the counsellor with additional techniques to use to resolve the difficulty in the session. There is far more material available than could possibly be taught in a five-day workshop and supervision is an opportunity to further the counsellor's skills.

A fully qualified and experienced counsellor has a variety of clinical skills to draw on if things do not go well and there is no immediate access to a supervisor. In our view, these additional clinical skills can be essential when working with a severely traumatized client. If a counsellor is not fully qualified and/or experienced then minimal supervision would not be appropriate. In our view 'fully qualified and experienced' means that the counsellor has training to work with more than one model and has worked with a variety of client groups. Extensive training in TIR and related methods is offered to counsellors who do not reach this level of expertise in some circumstances. Extensive training regimens usually include a closely supervised practicum of several months.

Use of TIR in Peer-Support Settings: A Word of Caution

Because of the strict definitions of roles and responsibilities for counsellors and clients in this method, it is possible to use TIR and related techniques in peer support settings where dual relationships might exist. In our opinion, this should be done very sparingly as issues of transference, and ability to disclose, often arise. We find that use of TIR as peer support, on a limited basis, is quite effective. During the experiential training workshop, we encourage people to use personal material in order to experience TIR from the client's perspective, and this works quite well.

Liberal use of case examples and case illustrations were used throughout this text and identifying details have been changed to protect these clients. Permission has been given to the authors to use these case illustrations.

The term 'counsellor' has been used for a variety of mental health professionals (including psychiatrists, psychologists, social workers, psychotherapists, peer support personnel, general practitioners and psychiatric nurses). Regardless of the number of degrees, diplomas or certificates held, or previous experience in the field of trauma work, training is strongly suggested for ALL mental health professionals who wish to adopt the methods detailed in this text when working with traumatized clients.

Non-sexist language   When appropriate, we used plurals in order to offend as few people as possible. In case examples, we remained true to the gender of the participants. In cases where plurals are awkward, we endeavoured to alternate between the use of male and female pronouns.

We have tried to define all new terms used in the text, and we strongly recommend the use of a dictionary for any words that the reader may find ambiguous.

AN OVERVIEW OF TRAUMATIC INCIDENT REDUCTION AS A BRIEF THERAPY APPROACH FOR POST-TRAUMATIC STRESS DISORDER

Traumatic Incident Reduction (TIR) was developed by an American psychiatrist, Frank Gerbode, in 1986. In this chapter we provide an overview of some aspects of the theory and an in-depth discussion of other aspects of the theory can be found later in the book. TIR is a directive, person-focused method of examining trauma. We are using the term *person-focused* instead of person-centred in order to distinguish our orientation from the school of person-centred counselling developed by Carl Rogers. To us, person-focused means that we consider any individual to be the expert on his own experience. He is the only one who can fully understand his experience – decide what it means, how it fits in the context of his own life and how it translates into his relationship with others. This is a central principle in TIR. We respect the client's own expertise and this informs our practice. We gain our information from our clients to help us guide them in examining their worlds in manageable pieces so that they can make sense of the whole.

The central concepts of TIR include: exposing the client to the trauma repeatedly, structuring the session closely, proceeding with work on a trauma or a group of related traumas in (preferably) one session until resolution (an end point) is reached. All related techniques in this model follow the same basic principles (which we examine in depth later in the book):

- Repetition as a way of facilitating the discharge of negative emotion and arriving at a cognitive shift – or insight.
- A non-judgemental and non-interpretive stance on the part of the counsellor (person-focused).
- Structured techniques that are made up of questions and instructions.
- Use of a defined end point (e.g. with specific criteria that depend on the process of the session rather than the content) to determine when to end the session. (An unfixed session time rather than a 50-minute or 90-minute session.)
- Use of specific communication skills.

THE STRUCTURE OF THIS BOOK

When we work with a client using these methods, we move through a variety of stages of treatment. This chapter provides an overview of each stage and illustrates the main technical skills involved in each stage of treatment. Chapter 2 provides an overview of the nature of Post-Traumatic Stress Disorder so that the reader has a framework in which to place the use of TIR as a brief therapy method. Chapter 3 provides an in-depth treatment of those clients who are suitable to benefit from TIR and related techniques as a brief therapy method for PTSD and discusses integrating TIR into longer term therapy in cases in which it would not be appropriate to use the model as a stand-alone method.

Chapter 4 provides an in-depth treatment of the first stage in brief therapy using TIR: the assessment and history-taking stage. This also includes further information about educating the client about the method. The second stage is the actual TIR work and is discussed in depth in Chapters 5, 6, 7 and 8. In the final stage, Chapter 9 provides a discussion of what to do when a TIR session does not go as planned, ending the counselling is discussed in Chapter 10. The appendices cover The Counselling Assessment Form (our history form), an Expanded Unblocking List and a graphical model of reaction to trauma. There are a variety of advanced techniques that we might use in more complex cases or situations, and these will form the subject of a separate book on Advanced Traumatic Incident Reduction.

RESEARCH ON TIR

There has been some controlled research on TIR as well as considerable anecdotal research that illustrates its efficacy as a treatment for PTSD (Bisbey, 1995; Coughlin, 1995; Figley, in press; Figley & Carbonell, 1995;

Gerbode, French & Van Aggelen, 1990; Gerbode, French & Bisbey, 1993). Treatment using TIR is usually short to medium term (under six months' treatment and often eight weeks' treatment) and intensive when possible. Controlled research results indicate that it is more effective than Direct Therapeutic Exposure, which is the most well-researched treatment of traditional methods (Bisbey, 1995) and that these results are maintained on follow up at six months, one year and two years (Bisbey, 1996a). In addition, anecdotal information sees treatment gains being maintained at five and eight years follow-up (Bisbey, 1996b).

LONG-TERM VERSUS SHORT-TERM WORK IN THE TREATMENT OF PTSD

There is considerable debate in the field of traumatic stress on the issues surrounding symptom resolution versus symptom management – sometimes described as remission versus cure. There are those who are convinced that symptoms can only be managed or that PTSD, once resolved, can become active in the face of other life circumstances. These clinicians and researchers subscribe to a disease model of PTSD similar to the models used in the substance abuse field. In our opinion, the largest problem with this model is that it cannot be either proved or disproved. When is PTSD seen as no longer 'in remission' but actually 'cured'? Is this after two years with no symptoms, four years, ten years?

Charles Figley, one of the most well-known experts in the field of traumatic stress, is one of the group who believes that it is possible to 'cure' or resolve* PTSD and that short-term treatment has proved to be quite successful in many cases (Figley, in press; Figley & Carbonell, 1995). We too believe, based on our experience and the research evidence, that it is possible to resolve PTSD. In this case, resolution is defined as the person no longer qualifying for a diagnosis of Post-Traumatic Stress Disorder. Depending on the circumstances, we feel that this is best done with short-term intensive treatment, particularly using TIR. We use a variety of cases to illustrate this throughout this book.

A variety of considerations have arisen regarding the benefits of long- versus short-term work. In Chapter 3, we discuss who is suitable for work with TIR (which is traditionally short to medium term). In brief, in situations in which a client has a limited ability to trust other human beings

---

* 'Cure' in this context means that the person no longer qualifies for a diagnosis of PTSD (or any other disorder that was caused by the trauma in question).

and a limited ability to communicate in relation to his thoughts and feelings, longer term treatment is usually necessary. In some cases, TIR is employed as part of a long-term treatment plan to address specific traumatic incidents and thematic material. In other cases, long-term treatment is done using related techniques and the same general theoretical constructs. In either of these situations, advanced techniques are necessary to enable the client to make use of the method. These are not covered in this book, but form the subject of a future book.

We recommend taking a holistic approach to the client, which is the reason we engage in such an in-depth history and assessment stage in our treatment. Some clients need additional treatment to learn new social skills, develop an identity that is not focused around the trauma, and learn to manage their intimate relationships – many of which have been impacted by the trauma. This is particularly true in cases of chronic Post-Traumatic Stress Disorder. In these cases, TIR can be integrated into a longer term treatment plan and, in addition, more advanced techniques can be applied which address these issues. Though we examine this briefly in Chapter 3, much of this is the subject of our book on Advanced Traumatic Incident Reduction.

In order for TIR to be successful, a client has to be able to tell the counsellor whatever might enter his mind, without censoring. This requires that the client must be able to trust the counsellor on quite a deep level. In addition, it requires the client to be able to communicate readily about thoughts and feelings. Some clients are unable to do this because they are not cognitively literate – e.g. they do not have the skill of introspection, and are often unable to verbalize thoughts and feelings except on a basic level. An example is one client who was asked what he was feeling at that moment and replied 'Nothing' while he was clenching his fists. When the counsellor probed this area, the client said, 'The only thing I feel is anger. I don't have words for feelings. I don't know how to describe these things.' Another example is of a client who, during a session, sat silently for a while and was asked by the counsellor what he was thinking at that moment. He replied, 'I don't know.' He then went on to tell the counsellor that he did not tend to think much and so was unable to tell the counsellor about his thoughts. With clients in this situation, the initial therapy focuses on developing trust in the therapeutic relationship and teaching the client how to identify and verbalize thoughts and feelings. Often the therapeutic relationship becomes the focus of the therapy as this relationship is different from previous relationships in the client's life.

When we teach workshops and give lectures on TIR, one of the areas frequently raised as a concern is whether or not the relationship between therapist and client is deep enough to do the work necessary. Trauma specialists frequently bring up the intensity of the material and the extreme importance of safety and trust in the therapeutic relationship. Many practitioners feel that short-term intensive work might not allow for a deep enough bond. Generally, this has not been our experience.

Because of the simplicity of TIR, the contact between therapist and client in a session can be extremely intense. As the practitioner places her full attention on her client, and she is not engaging in a discussion, making interpretations or judgements, there is no barrier between her client and herself during the session. When the emotion in the session becomes intense, she is right there in contact with the client and therefore in contact with the emotion and its intensity. This intensity can last quite a long time and therefore unfixed session times are essential to enable the client to get through it. As long as the counsellor consistently uses the specific communication skills and specific rules covered in this method of working, the client will feel safe in the session.

Because many sessions end on a positive note (as an end point has been reached), there is sometimes a feeling of elation for both the client and the therapist. For us, this type of session can best be described as a peak experience (using Maslow's definition). It is a time of great intimacy. Despite the shorter term nature of the work, in our experience, the intimacy is as deep as when working with clients on a long-term basis.

THE IMPORTANCE OF EXPOSURE IN WORKING WITH TRAUMA

In the field of trauma work, it is generally agreed that the methods that best enable a client to resolve traumatic experiences usually involve some form of exposure to the traumatic memories and the emotions, thoughts and sensations associated with these memories. By exposure, we usually mean that the client is asked to review the traumatic memory and talk about it, write about it, act it out or use art work to express the memory. Most forms of exposure-based work involve the client examining the memory in depth. In TIR, this exposure is accomplished through having the client review the trauma silently from beginning to end, and then tell the counsellor what happened. The client is asked to do this repeatedly until an end point is reached.

Gerbode calls the client, in TIR and related methods, a 'viewer' because he reviews the material contained in his mental environment (images, sounds, smells, tastes, sensations, feelings, thoughts). Gerbode calls the process 'viewing', which makes sense in this context. The viewing of the material provides the intensive exposure necessary for the client fully to process and make sense of the traumatic material that has not been integrated. Further theory on the nature of trauma is discussed in the next chapter.

In TIR, the use of repeated reviewing of the trauma allows the client to control his level of exposure to the trauma. He can control the intensity to some degree by contacting the traumatic material (including the often intense emotions) in stages. On each repetition, new details of the trauma may emerge, often the level of emotion (and the types of emotion) experienced changes, different aspects of the trauma are examined until insight is achieved and resolution occurs. At this point, the session ends. Integration of the trauma often happens during the session but can also happen in the days or weeks following the session.

Length of Exposure

As the client is exposed to the traumatic material, the emotions he experienced at the time of the trauma can be re-experienced in the session. Short exposure sessions usually only allow enough time for the emotion to reach its peak intensity. There is some evidence that ending a session when the emotion is at peak intensity only serves to retraumatize the client (Black & Bruce, 1989; Rothbaum & Foa, 1992). Part of the reason traumas are unresolved in the first place is that clients often feel that if they recontact those emotions, the negative emotions will overwhelm them and they will feel that way forever. They cannot conceive of experiencing the emotions and coming out of the session feeling better – and the emotions not recurring in the future. Consequently, exposure lengths must be long enough to allow the trauma to lose some of its emotional intensity. Ideally, they should be long enough for the trauma to lose *all* of its emotional intensity.

Many forms of exposure-based treatment use 90-minute session lengths instead of the classic 50-minute period. Ninety minutes was chosen because research on imaginal flooding (a behavioural exposure-based treatment) indicated that 90 minutes usually allows enough time for the emotion to reach its peak and then begin to drop significantly so that, at the end of the session, the level of negative emotion is less than it was at the beginning of the session, thus not retraumatizing the client (Rothbaum & Foa, 1992). Unlike TIR, this choice of length of session is still counsellor-focused rather than person-focused (e.g. it is chosen to fit into the counsellor's schedule rather than based on the client's process in the session).

End Points or Points of Closure in a TIR Session

In TIR sessions, the length of exposure is determined by the client's process and therefore the sessions are unfixed in length. This is a person-focused method of determining the length of session. Ideally, sessions are over when an end point is reached. Sometimes this is not possible, in which case the session is ended when a level place is reached.

An end point is the point at which the trauma (or group of traumas) being examined is considered to be resolved. There are specific factors that the counsellor must observe in the session before he considers the session to be at an end point. Most of these factors are process determined as opposed to content determined. Process factors look at the pattern of the session whereas content factors look at the details of what is said and expressed, or the presumed meaning or significance of what is said and expressed, during the session. The counsellor ends the session ideally when all three of the main criteria are met. The counsellor would not consider that an end point has been observed based on just one criterion.

The criteria for an end point in a session include:

Change in the client's emotional state in a strongly positive direction. This includes:

- A return of normal colour to the face.
- The client is laughing, smiling or demonstrating that he is feeling better.
- The client makes statements illustrating he is feeling better or feeling positive emotions such as feeling peaceful, feeling happy, the trauma has lost its intensity, the trauma no longer feels important.
- The client's body position indicates a more relaxed internal state.
- The client reports that negative physical sensations have disappeared.

The client's attention shifts from concentrating on his mental environment to an awareness of the external environment.

- The client makes sustained eye contact with the counsellor.
- The client notices things in the room.
- The client's attention turns to things in the physical environment (including feeling hungry, noticing the time, noticing external noises).
- The client comments on activities he will be involved in after the session (e.g., he is going to the gym after session, must make a call, has a meeting)
- The client comments on the counsellor or something about the counsellor.

There is evidence of a cognitive shift – the client's thinking about the meaning of the traumatic experience has changed.

- The client states that she has achieved insight into the experience.
- The client reframes the trauma in terms of a learning experience.
- The client makes connections between the trauma and other experiences in her life.
- The client reports that the trauma feels finished and is no longer as significant.
- The client reports that the experience now makes sense and talks about its meaning to her.
- The client loses interest in the trauma and in talking about the trauma.

A number of these signs must be present to consider that an end point has been reached. At this point, the counsellor ends the session. In some cases, these signs are not present but the client reports being tired, being hungry or being unable to go on – or the session has stagnated (the traumatic material and the client's view of this material is no longer changing). In these cases, the counsellor might end the session knowing that a full end point was not reached. Issues surrounding ending the session when there has not been a full end point are covered in Chapter 9.

We want to underline that these decisions are related to the process the client is involved in – working through the trauma – not specific content that the client expresses. We are not looking for *our* idea of an adaptive or significant resolution, we are looking for the *client's own* significant resolution. This is an important distinction as many counsellors, particularly those coming from a psychoanalytic background, are used to interpreting or reframing the client's statements of meaning relating to the trauma. In TIR work, we never do this; the client does it.

A Word about 'Negative' End Points

The causation of incidents comes in four directions which Gerbode refers to as 'flows'. These are:

1. *Victim*: Someone does something to traumatize the client. For example, a client is assaulted.
2. *Perpetrator*: The client does something that causes pain or trauma to someone else. For example, a soldier in war time kills a civilian.
3. *Witness*: The client witnesses a traumatic event. For example, the client sees a road fatality or witnesses physical violence between his parents.

4. *Reflexive*: The client causes something traumatic to happen to himself. For example, the client attempts suicide or drinks heavily and drives his car into a tree.

Most clients initially come in with traumas that are of the victim or witness type – things have happened to them or they have witnessed horrible things. Some clients are very traumatized by things they have done to others and they tend to examine perpetrator type traumas as well. (This is particularly true when the client has served in the military or in the police force.)

Because we do not interpret the client's experience, some counsellors have been concerned about clients coming to 'negative' or 'maladaptive' end points. For example, one counsellor who worked with perpetrators, was concerned that someone who had raped a person could use TIR to justify this action. Her concern was that in the process of examining the perpetration incidents, the client would come to the conclusion that his actions were justifiable or acceptable, and that because this was a cognitive shift, it would be accepted by the counsellor as part of an end point. She felt that if the session were ended at this point it would be validating the client's perception – that his actions were justifiable. In our experience, this type of situation does not arise because a client only tends to examine incidents that are personally traumatic to him – if the incident is not upsetting to him, he usually will not examine it. As a rule, TIR will not work with an incident that has no emotional or cognitive charge attached to it. So someone who had raped someone would only be willing to examine that incident if he had negative feelings about the incident, not just negative feelings about the consequences of the incident (e.g. arrest and jail time). For this reason, the insight at the end of a session is usually an objectively more adaptive one (e.g. the person who raped someone gains understanding as to why he did this and no longer feels a need to repeat this action or forgives himself for his action and now wants to do something to help the victim).

COMMUNICATION SKILLS AND RULES SPECIFIC TO TIR SESSIONS

Content of the insight (or cognitive shift) can be a controversial issue that is difficult for a counsellor and leads us into a discussion of what we mean by non-judgemental and non-interpretive – *person-focused* – work. In TIR and related work, we follow specific rules in addition to observing the regular ethical rules that most counsellors follow in their work. We also rely on high-quality communication skills during the session. These two factors (the rules we follow and the communication style we employ) are essential to creating a safe space for the client, one in which he will feel free to tell the counsellor whatever should cross his mind during the session.

During a TIR session as in other counselling sessions, the counsellor gains his information on the process of the session by noting the client's body language, noting the client's expression of emotion, and by what the client says. One difference between a TIR session and some other counselling sessions is that the counsellor is not making decisions based on the significance or meaning of the client's communication but rather on the type of communication. For example, if a client says that he is bored with the incident in a regular counselling session, this might be interpreted by the counsellor as avoidance of the emotion contained in the incident and usually the counsellor would express this to the client by saying something such as, 'Is it possible you are not bored but rather are finding this emotional material difficult to look at?' In a TIR session, the counsellor would not interpret but find out and consider the following possibilities if the client says he is bored with the incident:

1. There was no real interest in the incident to begin with – e.g. it was already resolved.
2. The counsellor has missed the end point which occurred earlier in the session.
3. There is no further charge in this incident, but other aspects of the incident need to be examined (such as cognitive content or an earlier connected incident).
4. The client is finding it difficult to look at the emotional material.

Note that these possibilities all relate to the process of the session. In a TIR session, the counsellor would have to find out from the client which of these possibilities is the most likely so that he could decide what to do to get the session moving towards a point of closure again. In order to find out, he would ask the client a variety of questions, such as, 'When did you start feeling bored with the incident?' The answer to that question helps the counsellor to rule out at least one of the four possibilities – that the material was not of interest in the first place. In addition, it could help the counsellor to determine if he had missed the end point earlier in the session. Based on the client's answer, the counsellor determines what to do next in the session. In order to make an accurate decision, the counsellor relies on the client being honest, and mentioning anything that comes to mind even if it does not seem related to the incident. As we said above, the client will not be willing to do this if he does not feel completely safe.

Aspects of Communication Necessary to Create Safety in a Session

One of the most important elements of communication necessary to create safety in a session is the counsellor's ability to remain non-judgemental and interested in the client regardless of what the client says or does. This does not mean the counsellor does not have her own normal human response to traumatic material. It means it is imperative that the counsellor keeps her attention firmly on the client and does not become distracted and move her attention to her own mental environment (such as thoughts, images, or feelings about what the client is saying). This seems an obvious concept but, in our experience, counsellors frequently spend considerable time during a session thinking about what they should do next, or reacting to what the client is saying rather than keeping in contact with the client.

Maintaining emotional contact with the client requires that the counsellor maintains interest in the client and what he is saying or doing. French and Gerbode (1995) define interest as directed attention. French points out that it is the client focusing his attention on an object that generates interest. It is not something inherent in the object that is interesting. Anything can be interesting if a person intentionally directs his attention towards it. Therefore interest is in the control of the person and can shift (e.g. something can be interesting at one point and not at another) rather than being an attribute of the object.

For example, suppose a counsellor goes to a wine-tasting party with a wine specialist. Both enjoy the party and discuss it afterwards. The wine specialist talks about how interesting the different types of wine were and talks with enthusiasm about their bouquets, flavours, body and smoothness. The counsellor talks about the interactions between the people at the party, their body language, conversation, displays of emotion and connection to others. The wine specialist is surprised as he did not notice the people at the gathering particularly – he was not interested in that aspect of the party. He did not pay attention to the interactions between the people. The counsellor enjoyed the wine but did not notice any of the fine distinctions between the different wines. His rating of the wines was based on much broader impressions – he either liked them or did not like them. His attention was focused on the people, finding them much more interesting.

This concept is important for two reasons. If the counsellor is not interested in the client, the client will not feel safe or inclined to fully engage in the session. If the counsellor becomes interesting to the client (e.g. the counsellor says or does something that draws the client's attention to the counsellor and away from the client's own material) then the client is not concentrating on his own material – which is his job in the session. When the counsellor is able to focus his full attention on the client, he is then able to stay in emotional contact with the client (because he is not distracted by his own mental environment). The counsellor then will not react *automatically* to the client's material and is less likely to distract the client with his own emotional reactions.

It is easier to be non-judgemental if the counsellor is not analysing the material the client is presenting. In analysing material, we relate it to our own feelings, thoughts, experiences, biases and attitudes and this makes it much harder to remain in emotional contact with the client. Analysis, if it occurs, should happen after the session, when the counsellor is free to shift her attention to her own mental environment. Systems of counselling which require the counsellor to pay attention to her own reaction to the client in the session (such as psychoanalysis) of necessity require less contact with the client during the session as one cannot give full attention to two things at once. This can result in the client feeling unsafe – because he feels the counsellor is not sufficiently interested in him or because he feels the counsellor is making emotional judgements about him as a person or about the material he is presenting.

During the TIR workshop, we spend some time doing exercises to help counsellors reinforce their skills in making and maintaining contact with clients in this non-judgemental way. In addition, the exercises help counsellors to hone their skills in asking non-interpretive questions.

In a TIR session, the counsellor does not make comments, suggestions or interpretations of the client's material. Instead, the counsellor uses good contact (e.g. maintaining full attention on the client), good acknowledgements and informed questions to establish safety, communicate empathy to the client, and guide the client in her own process (as opposed to being interesting and leading the client). French and Gerbode prefer the term 'facilitator' to the term counsellor for these reasons as they see a counselling role as implying the possibility of advice, suggestion and interpretation. They refer to the counsellor as a facilitator because that is what the counsellor does – he facilitates the client's process.

Acknowledgements are of two types: partial acknowledgements, which encourage the client to keep talking and let the client know the counsellor is listening and comprehending what he is saying; and full acknowledgements, which let the client know that the counsellor has heard and comprehended or understood what the client communicated. Because these acknowledgements are often short and to the point, session transcripts of a TIR session can seem quite sparse. Transcripts reproduced in this book will include asides that describe the emotional expressions and non-verbal communication from the counsellor and the client. However, the reader should remember that true contact with a client can be very emotionally intense and very difficult to describe in words. The actual feeling contained in the session is quite difficult to describe in a written format. Wherever possible, we will use quotes from clients and counsellors to illustrate this feeling and intensity.

All of the rules we use are designed to allow us to facilitate the process of the session rather than interrupt the process of the session. In order to demonstrate this, we ask that you try this exercise:

The next time someone wants to talk with you about something that is emotionally charged, see what happens if you listen to the person with your full attention (e.g. not thinking about what the person is saying and deciding what you will say next but rather continually redirecting your attention to the person and what he or she is saying) without interrupting, and when the person finishes, and before you answer acknowledge what the person has said by a short statement indicating that you have heard and understood (for example: 'fine' or 'OK'). Then compare this to what happens if you interrupt the person, make judgemental comments (such as 'I disagree' or 'I agree'), interpret the meaning of what the person says, or relate what he or she is saying to your own experience.

The primary rules we follow in TIR and related work are as follows. We have adapted these from Gerbode's (1990) Rules of Facilitation.* Some of them are obviously standard ethical principles followed by most counsellors. Others are specific to using TIR.

1. **The counsellor must not interpret for the client.**
   He must not tell the client what she is viewing or what it means. The client must be regarded as an authority on her own experience. It is understood from the outset, in the viewing process, that all statements made by the client are assumed to be prefixed by 'It is my opinion (or observation) that . . .'. Therefore the counsellor need not agree with the content of what is said; he simply agrees to accept the communication as a communication about the client's world.

2. **The counsellor must not evaluate for the client.**
   He must not attack, punish or invalidate the client or his ideas, perceptions or actions, *nor must he praise or validate them*. By 'evaluate' is

---

* We have replaced the terms 'facilitator' and 'viewer' with 'counsellor' and 'client' throughout.

meant suggesting in any way that the client is right or wrong for something she has said or done. This may require some skill on the part of the counsellor, since even a minor comment, grunt, gesture or change of facial expression can be interpreted as a sign of approval or disapproval. If the client feels threatened or made to feel wrong, her attention will be distracted to the counsellor, and she will no longer feel safe in the counselling session. Even if she is praised, the client may take this as an indication that the counsellor is judging her performance, and that the next judgement might not be so favourable.

3. **The counsellor must agree not to reveal or use anything the client says in a session for any purpose except with express permission of the client or for the purpose of supervision.**

4. **The counsellor must control the session and take complete responsibility for it without dominating or overwhelming the client.**

   This makes it unnecessary for the client to worry about controlling the session and allows him to put all of his attention on viewing. If he is concerned about what the agenda should be for the session, his attention will be distracted from its proper object: the material he is viewing. Conceptually, the counsellor is like a personal secretary or office manager who handles and screens all phone calls, keeps the files and reminds the executive of his appointments, so that the executive (in this case, the client) can do his job smoothly. Like a secretary, the counsellor keeps records of the session, keeps the agenda straight and reminds the client when he needs to take the next action. But it is the client who takes the action.

5. **The counsellor makes sure that he comprehends what the client is saying.**

   A client knows right away when she is not being comprehended. When that happens, she feels alone and unsupported. If the counsellor does not comprehend, she must seek clarification by admitting her lack of comprehension as something having to do with **her**, not the client. So she would say, 'I'm sorry – I did not understand what you said. Could you tell me again?' She would not say: 'You are being unclear', or 'That sounds like nonsense' or even 'Please clarify what you mean.'

6. **The counsellor must be interested in the client and what he is saying, instead of being interesting to the client.**

   If the counsellor becomes interesting, he will act as a distraction, pulling the client's attention to the counsellor instead of allowing the client to place her attention on the material she is examining. The counsellor's interest reinforces the client's willingness to view and report on the material she is examining. A client generally knows immediately whether or not the counsellor is really interested.

7. **The counsellor must ensure that the session is being given in a suitable space and at a suitable time.**
He or she ensures that the counselling environment is safe, private, quiet, a comfortable temperature and comfortably lighted. The counsellor also ensures that the **time** is safe. He makes sure that the client is not pressed for time and that suitable precautions have been taken against any need to interrupt the session for any reason.

8. **The counsellor should act in a predictable way so as not to surprise the client.**
If the counsellor engages in unpredictable actions, the client can become distracted by wondering what is going to happen next. This includes educating the client as to the way the counselling will proceed, what the counsellor will do in a session and what are his expectations of the client.

9. **The counsellor should not try to work with someone against that person's will or in the presence of any protest.**
Sometimes a relative or friend can persuade a person to attend counselling even when he does not really want to, or other pressures can be brought to bear on a person to attend counselling against his wishes. In such circumstances, trauma counselling does not work well, or at all. This includes insisting that the client examine a particular issue even when he has stated that it is not a problem for him or he has no interest in examining it.

10. **The counsellor must not do anything in a session that is not directly conducive to the counselling process.**
A counsellor who, during a counselling session, engages in social chit-chat, talks about himself, makes random comments, gives lectures or advice, laughs excessively or inappropriately, or indulges in emotional reactions towards the client, such as anger or expressions of anxiety, is distracting the client and often damaging the safe space. In this type of work, it has not proved effective for the counsellor to be 'honest' about his feelings to the client.

11. **The counsellor must finish what he starts and help the client to successfully conclude any step of the counselling programme.**
This includes having an open-ended session time so that sessions can continue to an end point for the client as well as returning to any areas that have not been completely resolved in a particular session in subsequent sessions.

Examples of violating these rules (and those specific communication rules used in this method) are given in Chapters 6 and 7.

OVERVIEW OF TIR PRACTICE

So far we have covered a brief description of the method of TIR, including the features common to all techniques based on this theory, a description of the research relating to TIR, a discussion of exposure and a discussion of the importance of the safe session space in TIR work. In this section, we will give an overview of the mechanics of an Unblocking session and a TIR session and a description of the types of additional questions a counsellor might use during the TIR session.

Unblocking

Unblocking is a technique that employs repetition to help a client fully examine a subject area or relationship until he gains some clarity and new insight. For some clients, it is an easier method than TIR because it does not require the client to contact a traumatic incident in its entirety and in all of its intensity. The technique consists of a list of questions, each of which is asked repeatedly until the client has no more answers to the question or until a point of closure is reached. The questions are built out of concepts that, in our opinion, constitute the types of intellectual defences a client employs which prevents him from having clarity about a given relationship or subject area.

Each time a question is asked, the client is encouraged to examine the area anew – looking at it from a different angle. It gives the client the opportunity to contact and express any emotion surrounding the area or relationship and to move past his own defences until he feels greater insight or the area is resolved. There are two lists of concepts – a short one and a long one. The longer one is usually used to examine more complex subject areas or relationships, such as a relationship with a parent. Counsellors are encouraged to develop their own questions from these lists – questions that will make sense to the client population with whom they are working. Sample questions and these lists are contained in Chapter 6 and Appendix 2.

Unblocking is used in a variety of situations. It is used when dealing with relationships in which there are so many potentially upsetting or traumatic incidents that would make it difficult to use TIR as a first step. TIR is more of a time-based linear technique – e.g., we examine groups of connected incidents in time moving from the most recent to those in the more distant past, whereas Unblocking is a more holistic technique addressing the thoughts and feelings of a subject regardless of the location in time of any events. Unblocking can be used when incidents of specific length (e.g.

with a beginning, a middle and an end) cannot be identified but a subject area or relationship is causing distress. For example, the client's job is causing a problem but he cannot identify specific incidents on the job that cause the problem.

Unblocking can be used before TIR to look at a specific trauma because the client can more easily manage the less intense contact with the incident. Unblocking is also used for incidents that lasted over a very long time period (such as a divorce process that lasted two years) where the client does not feel he can break the incident down into more manageable chunks. In these cases, separate incidents are often identified during the Unblocking and the counsellor switches to TIR during the same session. Unblocking can also be used after TIR on the same incident when an end point was reached but there are ramifications of the incident that have not been examined. For example, if a client was permanently injured in a car accident, this has current life consequences. The counsellor might choose to use TIR with the accident and any hospital treatment and then Unblock the accident to help the client examine the ramifications in his current life. An in-depth treatment of Unblocking (including specific instructions and examples) is found in Chapter 6.

Traumatic Incident Reduction

Traumatic Incident Reduction (TIR) comes in two forms: presenting incident and thematic. In presenting incident or basic TIR, we start with a defined known incident (such as a car accident, a miscarriage or an attack). In thematic TIR, we start with a feeling, a physical sensation or an attitude (such as a feeling of guilt, a pain in the neck or discomfort with men) that might be a part of many incidents. All incidents have themes going through them and themes that connect them to other incidents. Incidents can be associated because of similarities in content (such as two car accidents), environmental cues (such as a thunderstorm in two different incidents) and thematic connections (such as the same emotion in a number of incidents, or the same conclusion drawn from a number of incidents). What makes a session 'Basic' or 'Thematic' is where the client starts – from a specific incident or from a theme.

The basics of a TIR session involve having the client choose an incident to work on; identify and tell the counsellor when the incident happened and where it happened; identify and tell the counsellor how long the incident lasted; identify and tell the counsellor where he was at the time of the incident; find the beginning of the incident, review the incident from the beginning to the end in his mind, and then tell the counsellor what happened (which includes the story of the incident, the thoughts, feelings, sensations during the incident and the thoughts, feelings, sensations during the reviewing of the incident, and any associations or conclusions the client draws from this experience). The client is asked to review the incident repeatedly and tell the counsellor what happened until an end point is reached, his attention is drawn to an earlier incident or no further change (in content of the story, affect or thoughts about the story) occurs in the session. If an end point is reached, the counsellor ends the session. If the client's attention is drawn to an earlier incident, the counsellor directs the client to that incident and the process resumes with that incident. If there is no further change, the counsellor intervenes (usually in the form of asking a question, or asking the client to direct his attention to a specific aspect of the trauma on the next review – such as thoughts or feelings). The purpose of all interventions is to start the session moving again so that progress towards an end point can be continued.

In some cases, the client may examine a group (e.g. four or five) of connected incidents in the same session. In other cases, the client examines only one incident in the session. Connections between incidents are not necessarily readily apparent to the client or to the counsellor. It is important that the counsellor and the client accept whatever incident the client's attention is drawn to during the session – irrespective of whether the connection makes immediate sense. In our experience, by the time the client reaches an end point, the connection between the various incidents is obvious to him. It may still not be obvious to the counsellor, but this is not important as long as the criteria for an end point are fulfilled.

The specific instructions for basic and thematic TIR sessions are found in Chapter 7. The instructions for creating additional questions for use during the TIR session are found in Chapter 8.

2

THE NATURE OF POST-TRAUMATIC STRESS DISORDER

In the previous chapter we provided an overview of TIR and related techniques and issues surrounding their use with clients. In this chapter we examine the concepts that underpin stress, Post-Traumatic Stress Disorder and some of the theory of TIR. We cover the diagnoses associated with trauma (PTSD and Acute Stress Disorder) but it is important to remember that these are not the only disorders that develop as a result of trauma. For a more in-depth treatment of diagnosis, we suggest that readers study the *Diagnostic and Statistical Manual of Mental Disorders – IV* (American Psychiatric Association, 1994) as well as taking a workshop or course which covers the ethical use of these diagnoses.

We use some parts of these models to help educate our clients as to what to expect in counselling and to give a rationale for the type of counselling we engage in with them. Educating the client helps to increase cognitive literacy – the client's ability to introspect and express his thoughts and feelings in words. In this chapter we also illustrate some of this education process.

DEFINITIONS OF STRESS

In the past, the term 'stress' has been used to refer to the adaptive 'demands placed on an organism and to the organism's internal responses to such demands' (Coleman, Butcher & Carson, 1980, p. 105). To avoid confusion, Coleman and co-workers divide the concept into 'stressors', which are the adaptive demands (usually external), and 'stress', which is the effect (frequently maladaptive and internal) created within the organism by the 'stressors'. In our opinion, any text examining people's responses to extreme stressors, and how to treat these responses, must start by looking at stress as a general concept and people's responses to 'ordinary' stressors.

We all encounter stressors in our daily lives. These stressors come in a variety of types: physical, psychological and social. All types of stressors require us to adapt, and when we have difficulty adapting we experience this as stress. Stress can be experienced on a physical level – for example, when we catch a virus our bodies need to adapt. The virus is the stressor and our bodies' responses to it can be perceived as stress. If we are successful in adapting, we return to the status quo and our bodies have established a new defence (for example, antibodies to the particular virus). If we are not successful in adapting, our bodies continue to be stressed and move on to new attempts at coping with the stressor. We discuss physical stressors and the body's response more fully when we examine Selye's model later in the chapter.

Stress can be experienced on psychological and social levels, and the types of stressors and responses can vary considerably. The intensity in which we experience stress varies depending on a variety of factors. These include:

• The nearness of the stressor: e.g. are we anticipating a stressor in the near future?
• The perception of threat level of the stressor – including beliefs about our ability to cope.
• The stress tolerance of the individual.
• The availability of external resources and support.
• The number of stressors.
• The period of time over which the stressors occur.

Most people experience periods of heavy stress. Lazarus (1966) refers to these periods as a crisis and defines crisis as 'a limited period in which an individual or group is exposed to threats or demands which are at or near the limits of their resources' (p. 407). During a crisis, people are often challenged to develop new coping skills to come through the crisis and readjust. When this does not happen naturally, crisis intervention is a useful tool to help people develop these new coping skills and to return them to their normal pattern of functioning. Traumatic Incident Reduction can be a useful tool in crisis intervention as well as in the treatment of Post-Traumatic Stress Disorder when used shortly after a traumatic or stressful event.

Selye's Model

Hans Selye (1976) developed a model of biological reactions to continuing stressors. This model, the general adaptation syndrome, contains three stages of biological response. This model can be seen to parallel psychological response to continuing stressors as well. Selye's work is most often cited when looking at psychosomatic disorders (disorders in which psychological stressors cause physical responses leading frequently to physical illnesses).

Selye hypothesized that the body has a generalized defence system that is capable of warding off any form of stressor to which it might be subjected. He felt also that the body has localized systems which come into play at the sight of any localized injuries or infections and link into the generalized system. His generalized adaptation syndrome has three stages:

- Alarm reaction
- Resistance
- Exhaustion.

In the alarm reaction stage, the body sends out a 'call to arms of the defensive forces in the organism' (Selye, 1976, p. 36). At this point, the adrenal glands come into play. Once through the alarm stage, there is a stage of resistance in which the body actively combats the stressor and often symptoms disappear (or significantly diminish). If this does not succeed in combating the stressor and the body continues to be exposed over a period of time, then the exhaustion stage sets in. Ultimately, Selye felt that if the body were exposed for too long a period of time, death would eventually occur.

Selye worked on the biological principle that the body always tries to maintain homeostasis. Homeostasis is defined as 'the tendency of organisms to maintain conditions making possible a constant level of physiological functioning' (Coleman, Butcher & Carson, 1980, p. glossary IX). This concept also translates to psychological functioning. It has been our observation that people will attempt to maintain psychological conditions, social situations or relationships, and coping skills that will make it possible to keep a constant level of psychological or emotional functioning. When stressors interfere with this constant (or normal) level of functioning, the person will put into action strategies to return to homeostasis as soon as possible. In some cases, the person will maintain maladaptive coping strategies in an effort to maintain homeostasis. In these cases, some type of therapy or counselling is often necessary to help the person to shed maladaptive strategies in favour of more adaptive ones.

Williams (1986) developed a model of response to trauma based on Selye's model. Williams' model is often used in psychological debriefing and crisis intervention after trauma to help educate clients about normal responses. We have adapted this model for use in the same situations, and our adaptation can be found in Appendix 3.

Selye also formulated the concept of eustress* versus distress. Selye postulated that people would have the same physiological reactions to stressors perceived as positive as they would to stressors perceived as negative. In his research, he discovered that this was correct but that when things were perceived as positive, the return to homeostasis or to a new stronger way of functioning was much more rapid than when a stressor was perceived as negative. He referred to positive stressors as *eustress* and negative ones as *distress*. When looking at life stressors, examples of eustressors include getting married, getting a promotion at work, moving to a new and better house, and having a child; examples of distressors include divorce, death of a loved one, losing a job and failing at something important to the person. Selye pointed out (and others have since confirmed) that people can become more susceptible to physical illness when there are a variety of eustressors as well as when there are a variety of distressors.

This model seems to apply to psychological reactions as well. We have observed that people seek out challenges and when there is not an adequate balance of challenge (eustress) in their lives, there is a tendency for negative situations (distress) to arise. In addition, it is important to consider the effects of eustressors as well as distressors when looking at sources of stress for any given individual at any given time. The symptoms experienced can be a result of a combination of eustress and distress rather than just a result of distress. We have frequently observed this in our practice. Positive events bring with them many challenges and sometimes call into question existing ways of coping and existing skills.

A User-Friendly Definition of Stress

Stress, as we define it, occurs when external demands and/or internal demands, or a combination of both, exceed the person's normal ability to cope and to maintain his or her ordinary function. Note that this definition allows for stress experienced as the result of 'ordinary' life stressors and critical or traumatic events. We will now move on to a discussion of traumatic and critical incidents.

---

* Eustress is defined as stress that occurs as the result of a perceived positive situation or event.

THE NATURE OF TRAUMA

Developments in cognitive psychology provide considerable insight into how trauma affects someone using explanations based on information-processing models. In a simplified form these models can be used to educate clients in the theories of how traumas impact the way they do in terms of recognizable mental phenomena.

When the brain is thought of as an information-processing system, a trauma can be described as an overwhelming input of information of sufficient magnitude to bypass an individual's capacity to selectively direct his attention. Selective attention is easily demonstrated for a client by having him selectively pay attention to the various sights, smells and noises in the counselling room and then to his own internal physical sensations, feelings and thought processes. His information-processing system can be further demonstrated by inviting him to become aware of his recognition of the environmental stimuli in his physical and mental environments and realize that this is a processing activity. (The comparison of incoming information to information already stored in memory enables recognition and then articulation.)

The idea of limited mental capacity (Broadbent, 1954) can be demonstrated by inviting the client to try to absorb all the sights, sounds and feelings she can be aware of at once. Dividing attention in this way inevitably means that not all incoming communication can be consciously processed. Treisman (1960) improved on Broadbent's (1954) attention theory to show that, even when attention is paid to a particular channel of incoming information, unattended channels are perceived and recorded, albeit unconsciously. Experiments by Neisser (1967) showed that visual inputs were automatically recorded without the necessity for conscious processing, and since then much research has been conducted which illustrates just how much information processing goes on at an automatic level.

In everyday experience, the automatic processing of data can be conceived as made possible by the existence of mental schemata (an idea introduced by Bartlett, 1932). A schema (or schemata) is a hypothesized mental structure constructed over time which categorizes knowledge and experiences recorded in memory. Once constructed, a schema's function is not only passive, encoding new information and aiding retrieval of it, but also active, in explaining or interpreting new data or experience pertinent to the schema (which then updates and modifies it). Data or experience for which an individual has no pre-existing schema requires the creation of an entirely new schema which, if it contradicts an old one, may be experienced as confusing or traumatic.

For example, an experienced driver can navigate from home to work using very little conscious attention to the driving or the route because prior learning has established mental schemata that enable the activity to be accomplished virtually automatically. In modern cognitive theory, such schemata can be conceived as neural networks in parallel distribution models (McClelland and Rumelhart, 1986). Networks are established through everyday learning experiences, which then facilitate the processing of incoming information.

When an individual is faced with having to engage in a new activity for which he has no pre-established schemata or neural network, considerably more conscious attention has to be directed to the activity. Driving a route for the first time is an example. When a person's limited mental capacity is stretched, such as driving a new route in icy conditions, stress may be experienced. When mental capacity is exceeded and attention can no longer be selectively directed – in the event of a car accident perhaps – then serious stress or trauma can result. Firstly, the quantity and quality of incoming information cannot be consciously processed and, secondly, there may be no 'car accident' schemata or neural network to assimilate and make sense of it. Compounding the trauma would be the contradiction created by schemata activated prior to the trauma. In this example, the individual's expectations (cognitive script) might minimally include the idea that cars are safe and move in the direction in which they are steered and stop when braked; that a journey to work will result in arriving at work. In other words, prior thinking, security, confidence, experience and expectations become invalidated.

Part of the definition of trauma has been 'abnormal experience'. In cognitive terms, 'abnormal', for an individual, would mean no pre-existing schemata or neural network capable of assimilating and accommodating that experience. The ongoing process of learning that establishes the schemata or neural networks capable of assimilating and accommodating further learning experience generally occurs gradiently and with conscious attention within an individual's mental capacity. A learning experience that exceeds an individual's mental capacity could be characterized as 'conditioning' when pre-existing schemata are invalidated and new schemata are established that have not been subject to adequate conscious analytical inspection and evaluation.

Such an experience is therefore always stressful and likely to result in symptoms of an acute stress reaction (or Acute Stress Disorder as discussed later in the chapter). If an individual automatically brings his other knowledge and experience (schemata or parallel neural networks) and assimilates and accommodates the experience, it can move into long-term memory and normal mental functioning is re-established. If not, the new unintegrated schemata or neural network can remain active or capable of continual activation by environmental cues until it is integrated. The result of this is Post-Traumatic Stress Disorder, a consequence of the functional and adaptive quality of the mind in that it demands that incoming information is processed and allocated to its appropriate schematic slot.

This phenomenon can be demonstrated to clients by asking them to recall times when they encountered something they did not understand and then made sense of it. A word they did not understand, an event in the street they had to satisfy themselves about, a physical sensation – anything they encountered for which they had no meaning. In each case, processing has to occur in response to the input, even if it is to ignore it.

Using the cognitive model, the treatment of trauma becomes a process of enabling the client to do what she was unable to do at the time of the traumatic experience – i.e. consciously attend to the inputted information that has been recorded but not inspected or evaluated. Pre-existing schemata may need to be re-evaluated and modified to accommodate and assimilate the new ones. PTSD is a comparative state by definition, the abnormal experience contrasting with the normal and having created abnormal symptoms. The condition rests and depends upon what went before and therefore the beginning of the incident is not necessarily the moment of the car crash but the pre-existing condition, schemata and cognitive script. This is reflected in the way in which clients use TIR. Sometimes, clients place the beginning of the incident days or even weeks before the specific incident occurred. For example, a client who was in a road traffic accident after spending the evening in the pub, placed the beginning of the incident at the beginning of the evening when he began drinking because he felt that if he had not been drinking, he would not have had the accident. Another client who was attacked started examining the incident from earlier in the day when she was looking forward to going out that evening. However, in most cases, as one might expect, clients identify the beginning of a trauma as the moment a stressor impacted upon them. The context in which it happened and prior schemata often are not taken into account.

In trauma counselling, the person-focused point of view is essential because the counsellor begins with no idea of what is normal for that particular client, i.e. what his prior schemata contain. History taking provides lots of clues. Additionally, it has been our experience that what we expected to find as traumatic sometimes turned out not to be, and what was traumatic was something less predictable. For example, a former professional soldier blown up by a terrorist's bomb identified his trauma as the way he behaved *afterwards* (e.g. when he went into shock) which was in contrast to his lifelong schemata of his self-image and professional identity and not the incident itself, which had provided an opportunity for heroism. In this case, the information contained in the memory of the obvious 'trauma' (the bomb blast) hardly needed any conscious processing in counselling. It was merely the precipitating factor for what happened in the days that followed. In the education of clients, the information-processing model can be a useful explanatory model, particularly if it fits in with their previous understanding or schemata!

DEFINITION OF TRAUMATIC AND CRITICAL INCIDENTS

As underlined in the previous section, it is important that any definition trauma counsellors use for traumatic and critical incidents in clinical practice is person-focused. There are a variety of definitions relating to traumatic and/or critical incidents in use in psychology at the present time. For an in-depth treatment of the subject, we suggest the reader sees such standard texts as *Trauma and Its Wake*, Vols 1 and 2, edited by Charles Figley, and *Human Adaptation to Extreme Stress: From the Holocaust to Vietnam* edited by John Wilson, Zev Harel and Boaz Kahana. We will give an overview of some common definitions leading to the definitions that we use in working with TIR and related methods of working.

The *Diagnostic and Statistical Manual of Mental Disorders – III Revised*, in its definition of a traumatic event qualifying for the diagnosis of Post-Traumatic Stress Disorder, states that the person must experience an event that is 'outside the range of ordinary human experience' (American Psychiatric Association, 1987, p. 250). This includes witnessing horrific events as well as participating in them. This definition, which is still used by quite a number of people working in the field, was revised in the *Diagnostic and Statistical Manual of Mental Disorders – IV* to read 'the person experienced, witnessed, or was confronted with an event or events that involved actual or threatened death or serious injury, or a threat to the physical integrity of others' and 'the person's response involved intense fear, helplessness, or horror' (American Psychiatric Association, 1994, pp. 427–428). We will not argue the merits (or lack thereof) of this change in diagnostic definition here. There were a variety of reasons for the change, not the least of which was the increase in litigation relating to traumatic incidents.

French and Gerbode (1995) propose the following definition of a traumatic incident: 'An incident that is wholly or partially repressed and that contains a greater or lesser degree of pain – felt, created, or received – and charge (repressed, unfulfilled intention).' While we agree with this definition because it is person-focused and defines a phenomenon without judgement, we propose a more user-friendly definition. In our view a trauma is **any event or experience that is outside the person's usual or ordinary experience and expectations about the way in which the world works and/or the way in which people treat each other**.

We must stress again that in terms of treatment with TIR (or any method of trauma counselling for that matter), counsellors must use a person-focused definition rather than a diagnostic one in helping to determine which incidents it might be fruitful to address. The DSM diagnostic definition is important in terms of treatment outcome research, determining potentially effective treatments, education of practitioners (and discussion among practitioners), possibly prevention and certainly in litigation, but if one stuck to a purely diagnostic definition in defining trauma, then one would lose site of the issues that are important to individuals and miss out on the opportunity to help in a variety of circumstances. TIR is extremely effective with events that, while not defined as traumatic incidents by a diagnostic definition, do qualify as a trauma for the individual involved. For example, we frequently use TIR in situations where someone has been bereaved. Certainly 'ordinary' bereavement (such as due to old age) does not fit in as a qualifying incident in the diagnostic definition. It is, however, frequently personally traumatic and bears looking at. Another 'common' event that fits this is miscarriage. This is frequently a very traumatic experience for the individual and sometimes produces the symptoms of Post-Traumatic Stress Disorder but in and of itself is not a qualifying trauma for the diagnosis as per the DSM.

DIAGNOSES PERTAINING TO STRESS

There are two diagnoses pertaining to stress: Acute Stress Disorder and Post-Traumatic Stress Disorder. Acute Stress Disorder is defined by the *Diagnostic and Statistical Manual of Mental Disorders – IV* (1994, pp. 431–432) as follows:

A. The person has been exposed to a traumatic event in which both of the following were present:
  (1) the person experienced, witnessed, or was confronted with an event or events that involved actual or threatened death or serious injury, or a threat to the physical integrity of others
  (2) the person's response involved intense fear, helplessness, or horror.

(*continued on p. 28*)

(*continued from p. 27*)
B. Either while experiencing or after experiencing the distressing event, the individual has three (or more) of the following dissociative symptoms:
    (1) a subjective sense of numbing, detachment, or absence of emotional responsiveness
    (2) a reduction in awareness of his or her surroundings (e.g., 'being in a daze')
    (3) derealization
    (4) depersonalization
    (5) dissociative amnesia (i.e., inability to recall an important aspect of the trauma).
C. The traumatic event is persistently reexperienced in at least one of the following ways: recurrent images, thoughts, dreams, illusions, flashback episodes, or a sense of reliving the experience; or distress on exposure to reminders of the traumatic event.
D. Marked avoidance of stimuli that arouse recollections of the trauma (e.g., thoughts, feelings, conversations, activities, places, people).
E. Marked symptoms of anxiety or increased arousal (e.g., difficulty sleeping, irritability, poor concentration, hypervigilance, exaggerated startle response, motor restlessness).
F. The disturbance causes clinically significant distress or impairment in social, occupational, or other important areas of functioning or impairs the individual's ability to pursue some necessary task, such as obtaining necessary assistance or mobilizing personal resources by telling family members about the traumatic experience.
G. The disturbance lasts for a minimum of 2 days and a maximum of 4 weeks and occurs within 4 weeks of the traumatic event.
H. The disturbance is not due to the direct physiological effects of a substance (e.g., a drug of abuse, a medication) or a general medical condition, is not better accounted for by Brief Psychotic Disorder and is not merely an exacerbation of a preexisting Axis I or Axis II disorder.

Post-Traumatic Stress Disorder is defined by the *Diagnostic and Statistical Manual of Mental Disorders – IV* (1994, pp. 427–429) as follows:

A. The person has been exposed to a traumatic event in which both of the following were present:
    (1) the person experienced, witnessed, or was confronted with an event or events that involved actual or threatened death or serious injury, or a threat to the physical integrity of others
    (2) the person's response involved intense fear, helplessness, or horror.
B. The traumatic event is persistently reexperienced in at one (or more) of the following ways:
    (1) Recurrent and intrusive distressing recollections of the event, including images, thoughts, or perceptions. *Note*: In young children, repetitive play may occur in which themes or aspects of the trauma are expressed.
    (2) Recurrent distressing dreams of the event. *Note*: In children, there may be frightening dreams without recognizable content.

(3) Acting or feeling as if the traumatic event were recurring (includes a sense of reliving the experience, illusions, hallucinations, and dissociative flashback episodes, including those that occur on awakening or when intoxicated). *Note*: In young children, trauma-specific reenactment may occur.

(4) Intense psychological distress at exposure to internal or external cues that symbolize or resemble an aspect of the traumatic event.

(5) Physiological reactivity on exposure to internal or external cues that symbolize or resemble an aspect of the traumatic event.

C. Persistent avoidance of stimuli associated with the trauma and numbing of general responsiveness (not present before the trauma), as indicated by three (or more) of the following:

(1) efforts to avoid thoughts, feelings, or conversations associated with the trauma

(2) efforts to avoid activities, places or people that arouse recollections of the trauma

(3) inability to recall an important aspect of the trauma

(4) markedly diminished interest or participation in significant activities

(5) feeling of detachment or estrangement from others

(6) restricted range of affect (e.g., unable to have loving feelings)

(7) sense of a foreshortened future (e.g., does not expect to have a career, marriage, children, or a normal life span).

D. Persistent symptoms of increased arousal (not present before the trauma), as indicated by two (or more) of the following:

(1) difficulty falling or staying asleep

(2) irritability or outbursts of anger

(3) difficulty concentrating

(4) hypervigilance

(5) exaggerated startle response.

E. Duration of the disturbance (symptoms in Criteria B, C, and D) is more than one month.

F. The disturbance causes clinically significant distress or impairment in social, occupational, or other important areas of functioning.
  Specify if:
Acute: if duration of symptoms is less than 3 months
Chronic: if duration of symptoms is 3 months or more
  Specify if:
With delayed onset: if onset of symptoms is at least 6 months after the stressor.

CLIENT'S DESCRIPTIONS OF THESE SYMPTOMS

Intrusion Symptoms

Description of flashbacks:

It was like I was back there again – in the middle of it. Suddenly I felt as if my husband were my father and I had to stop him in the middle of making love – open my eyes and check to make sure it was my husband. I had to look at his face

– and sometimes, that didn't do it and we had to stop completely because I felt as if his hands on me were my father's hands. On one level, I was aware of where I was and who I was with – but the feeling was just so overwhelming that it didn't matter.

Description of intrusive imagery:

I can be talking with friends about a new movie or book and suddenly his face will be there. Or I'll get a flash of him on top of me. I can be watching television – a comedy or something and suddenly I will see his face or body or I'll hear his voice. It is frightening and I can't concentrate.

Avoidance Symptoms

Description of a sense of foreshortened future:

I just know I won't have children or get married. I just won't be around that long. It's not like I want to kill myself or will do myself harm. It's just knowing that I'm not going to live a long life. I won't die of old age. I don't know what I'll die of – but I won't make it past 40.

Description of avoidance symptoms:

I won't watch anything on television to do with rape, crime victims or crime – which means I don't watch the news because I can never be sure what will be on it. I don't read newspapers either. I used to be an informed person but now I rarely know what is going on in current events. Its embarrassing but I cannot bring myself to watch the news or read the paper because I might get upset and that would be even more embarrassing. I feel different from people around me, separate and distant. Its like watching yourself go through your life – not really involved, not really there.

Arousal Symptoms

Description of hypervigilance:

I have to know where the doors are all the time – in any room. I have to know how I will get out. It is like having eyes in the back of your head – always being aware when someone moves behind you – always being on edge. Being exhausted all the time.

Description of hypervigilance:

Whenever I go into a pub, I can tell who was over there (Northern Ireland). They are all standing so they can see the rest of the room. All of us are aware of who is walking behind us and what is going on around us. We are tuned to any noises or sudden movements – to look for unusual boxes and cases or anything that seems out of place. It's like having radar – or antennae – constantly scanning the environment in case anything is amiss.

Dissociative Symptoms

Description of derealization:

Nothing seems real – it all seems like a movie going on around me. People seem to be two dimensional. It's a strange feeling. Like going in slow motion.

Description of depersonalization:

You'll think I'm mad if I tell you about this. It feels like I am separate from myself – a different person, watching myself go through things but not really being me. I'm like watching myself from a distance. And I think things like, 'Now she's going to do that. Now she's going to pick up the brush and brush her hair.'

Description of depersonalization:

I went away somewhere in my head, like I knew what was going on, but I wasn't really there. It was the oddest feeling. I could see myself being bounced around and I knew it must hurt but it didn't hurt because I was watching it and not really there.

Description of dissociation:

I left my body and was floating above myself looking down and watching the accident happen. I could see the cars crash and then could see myself being thrown from the car. I could see the ambulances pull up and see them lifting me onto the ambulance. They were talking to me but it was like I was very far away. I couldn't feel anything. Then, all of a sudden I was back in my body and I hurt badly.

Description of dissociation:

I was up on the ceiling. I could see the doctors operating on me on the table, but I was watching from the ceiling. I could hear the doctor say 'My god, there's a lot of scarring there. These tonsils were abscessed for a long time. She must have been in a lot of pain.' Then I was asleep again. When I woke up after the surgery, I checked with the doctor and asked if he had said that the tonsils had been abscessed. He was very surprised and admitted he had said that. When I told him I had watched the whole thing from the ceiling, he didn't believe me.

THEORETICAL MODEL OF TIME AND ATTENTION: THE NATURE OF PTSD FOR THE CLIENT

Gerbode's Model: The Nature of Time

Gerbode suggests that each individual has a limited amount of potential intention (defined as attention plus volition) or mental energy available at any one time. Gerbode postulates that though time is seen as a 'never-ending stream', subjectively it is actually experienced as divided into finite periods and these periods are defined by whatever activity is going on at the time. For example, one can speak of 'the time when I was

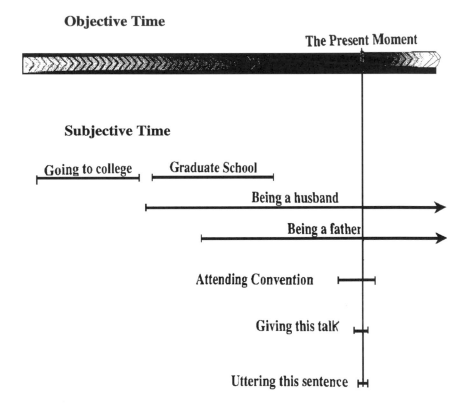

Figure 1: Objective time versus subjective time. Objective time is perceived as a never-ending stream. Subjective time is defined by where we choose to place our attention at any given moment. (Reproduced by kind permission of F. Gerbode, 1993.)

engaged to be married' or 'when I was in graduate school' as representing finite periods of time. The present can be perceived as subjectively
longer or shorter depending on the activities one chooses to use to define
it (Figure 1).

All activities have a beginning, a middle, and an end (Figure 2). This is
referred to as a cycle. A cycle begins when a person formulates an intention to either do (creative action) or be aware of (receptive action) something. The cycle continues until the person no longer has that intention.
For example, suppose that person A intends to read a book on the nature
of time. Person A has started a cycle when he formulates the intention.
The cycle continues until he has fulfilled that intention and has finished
reading the book or until he changes that intention by deciding to do
something else or deciding not to read the book at all.

If an individual does not complete an activity and still has the intention to
complete it, the cycle continues and some intention remains devoted to
that unfinished cycle. Therefore, the cycle continues into the present. The
present consists of all the cycles that are currently ongoing. Subjectively,
if one has too many unfinished cycles, one cannot begin new cycles.

Intention: Understand the nature of time

Activity: Read a book on the nature of time

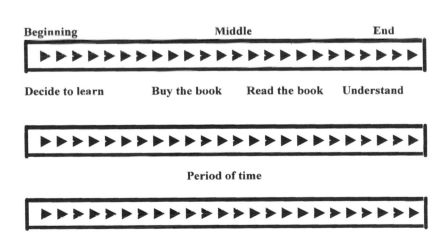

Figure 2: Intention and time

When an unresolved or traumatic incident occurs, some of an individual's attention becomes trapped in that situation or in the continued action of repressing that situation. It also takes some attention to avoid thinking of something or allowing a thought or image to come into consciousness.

Obviously, one then has less attention to devote to current pursuits or to use in handling current situations. When most of a person's attention is trapped in unfinished cycles of the past, he is said to be living in the past, rather than the present (Gerbode, 1989). Research with concentration camp survivors supports the idea that major trauma can cause a person to continue to live in the past and to be unable to orient himself towards the present or the future (Lomranz, Shmotikin, Zechovoy & Rosenberg, 1986). Lomranz and co-workers, found that this disability caused many problems for the subjects in their current lives. The study contained 75 subjects, 44 of whom were concentration camp survivors and 31 of whom made up a control group. Subjects were asked to complete two measures, The Life Line and the Time Orientation Questionnaire. The results indicated that, compared to the control group, subjects in the survivor group felt that the Holocaust time period was significantly closer to their present and a majority of the survivors could not set an end point to the time period as they felt it still continued into the present. In addition, survivors were found to be significantly more past oriented than the control group.

It takes a certain amount of energy to deal with any given situation, day-to-day. When a person does not deal with a situation but rather represses or dissociates it, he must keep some attention in that area to keep the disturbing material out of awareness. These concepts are similar to Freud's ideas of the finite amount of libido, Sullivan's theory of selective inattention and very close to Broadbent's ideas of limited mental capacity, as described earlier in this chapter.

The Traumatic Incident Network

According to Gerbode, each individual has a traumatic incident network (Figure 3). It helps if one can visualize the network as a tree with the earliest incidents as the roots, and sequences of incidents forming the trunk and branches (Figure 4). A root incident may be the beginning of many sequences or branches or a particular branch may have many roots. The incidents closer to the present are either in awareness or closer to awareness and often the root incidents are repressed or partially repressed.

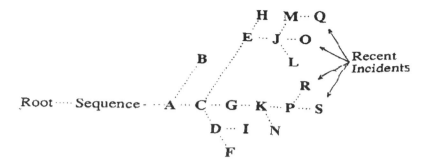

Figure 3: Traumatic Incident Network. Recent incidents from sequences which connect to root incidents. In this case, the letters represent incidents all leading back to the root, incident A. (Reproduced by kind permission of F. Gerbode, 1990, p. 112.)

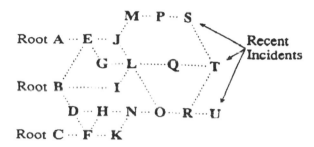

Figure 4: Traumatic Incident Network. This illustrates the tree structure of the network with multiple roots (incidents A, B, C) (Reproduced by kind permission of F. Gerbode, 1990, p. 113.)

New incidents on a sequence are created each time something happens that threatens to bring earlier incidents or the root incident into awareness. Each time this occurs, a certain amount of energy or 'charge' is added to the incident to help keep it repressed. Gerbode defines 'charge' as 'repressed, unfulfilled intention' (Gerbode, 1989, p. 505). Unless the incident is dealt with and its 'charge' reduced, the incident can be re-awakened and the feelings from the incident can be reawakened (triggered) repeatedly in various situations. In practice, charge often refers to the unresolved negative emotions contained in the incident that are triggered which results in the entire incident being triggered.

For example, suppose a 1-year-old child is accidentally scalded by hot water when being bathed by the sitter who wore a paisley dress, had grey hair and smelled like rubbing alcohol. The scalding becomes a root incident and contains primary pain. Primary pain is actual physical pain or

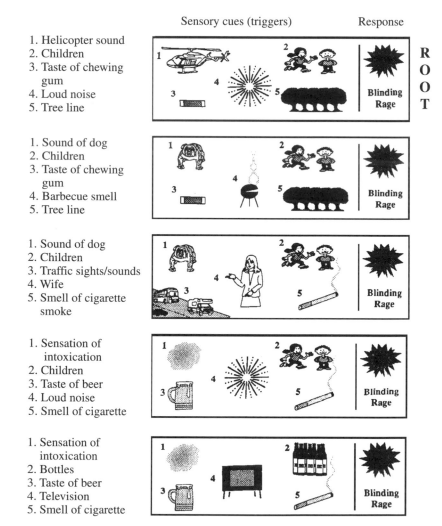

Sensory cues (triggers)   Response

1. Helicopter sound
2. Children
3. Taste of chewing gum
4. Loud noise
5. Tree line

1. Sound of dog
2. Children
3. Taste of chewing gum
4. Barbecue smell
5. Tree line

1. Sound of dog
2. Children
3. Traffic sights/sounds
4. Wife
5. Smell of cigarette smoke

1. Sensation of intoxication
2. Children
3. Taste of beer
4. Loud noise
5. Smell of cigarette

1. Sensation of intoxication
2. Bottles
3. Taste of beer
4. Television
5. Smell of cigarette

Figure 5: A sequence of traumatic incidents. Note the root at the top is the original incident. Note also that the response is a theme that runs through all of the incidents. (Reproduced by kind permission of G. French and F. Gerbode, 1995, p. 67.)

situational pain (extreme emotional upset attached to the situation) that is not derived from the triggering of an earlier incident. At the time of the incident, the baby is unable to confront the pain and negative emotion and so partially represses it.

A year later the toddler is told off by a woman in a paisley dress and becomes extremely upset. The toddler is reminded of the scalding incident and becomes even more upset. The first or root incident is said to be triggered; that is, the child experiences the emotions from both the initial incident and the current incident. It may be that the child would have been less upset had the telling off not reminded him of that earlier incident which was out of awareness.

At this time, the child can do one of two things: the child can confront both incidents, experience and discharge the emotions from them, engage in cognitive restructuring and so resolve them, thus ending the cycle that began with the scalding, or the child can repress or partially repress both incidents. If the child partially represses or fully represses both incidents, any element of either incident can potentially become a trigger for the whole sequence of incidents. (See, for example, the sequence in Figure 5.)

Gerbode suggests that what frequently holds a sequence of incidents in place is the intention the person had, or decisions the person made, at the time of the incident. These thoughts are often repressed and the person continues to carry them forward into his current life.

CLIENT EXAMPLES OF TRIGGERING OF THE TRAUMATIC INCIDENT NETWORK

Case 1: Mary, sexual abuse in childhood:

Sometimes I have to stop in the middle of having sex with my husband and open my eyes to make sure that it is him.

Joe, trauma following the break up of two marriages:

I will be talking with Wendy and she will say something, the tone of her voice or the expression on her face and all of a sudden I will call her Carol. It's like being in the middle of an argument with Carol. I won't realize it at the time. Usually I don't realize it until Wendy points it out to me.

The scent of a particular perfume, Chanel, I think will trigger me as well. I can be in a perfectly good mood and smell this perfume and then I will get angry and snap at whoever is there.

Paul, PTSD following armed police service:

I cannot be around fireworks. Every time I hear the bang, I am sure that people are shooting. I can be aware that it is fireworks on one level, but cannot prevent myself from startling and looking for cover.

THE NATURE OF TRAUMA

There may be any number of elements that serve to hold a trauma in place in the present, as an ongoing experience, rather than letting it fall into a historical perspective. It is the job of the counsellor to discover what these are when a client cannot discover them for herself. In addition to sensory cues (conscious and unconscious sights, sounds, smells), there are a variety of other triggers that a counsellor can explore.

1. Environmental Triggers

These might seem obvious but are easily overlooked, especially by a traumatized person. They might include:

A. *Intimates, friends and family asking about the client's experience*

When a person has a good support system, then these people will take a great interest in the trauma and in how the client is doing. Whereas support is extremely important, it is often the case that other people are more interested in the event or the story and do not afford a person the opportunity to process what actually went on in her own mental environment. Instead (naturally), a person will tend to construct her own *script* for people, a *version* of the event that is calculated (albeit unconsciously) to be palatable to her audience. This version might well be modified according to the person's social situation at the time.

For example, a man who was mugged by two people might well create a script for his girlfriend that added inches in height and extra weight to his attackers, added efforts to deal with the situation and minimized the shock of it. In another example a rape victim might minimize the full extent of the horror of the attack while talking to her mother about it. In effect a person will tend to create a version of events in deference to his audience. It is this editing that necessitates counselling. In counselling (hopefully), the client can process the *entire real* experience without worrying about the person who is listening. Nevertheless, whatever version of the trauma is being discussed, every time its script is described the trauma is kept alive. If it is an edited version of events, then it has limited value as far as discharging it and resolving it is concerned.

B. *Media*

Everywhere they look, traumatized people often appear to find newspaper articles and television programmes that somehow relate to their trauma. It is not that people consciously look for them. Their attention, caught up in and focused on the trauma, notices incoming information presented to them. Clients are usually aware of this type of triggering.

C. *Avoidance behaviour*

This can either be conscious or unconscious and consists of the traumatized person avoiding 'triggers' that might remind him of the event. Some of them might be obvious and known to the client – for example, not going back to the Post Office where he was mugged. Others may be a little more subtle – for example, an unconscious avoidance of documentary programmes on crime.

Avoidance behaviour as well as being a symptom of trauma, actually adds to it. Attention is needed to avoid a location, a person, a trigger of whatever kind. This serves to keep the trauma in the present.

D. *Legal and other consequences*

On many occasions a trauma can mean that it is necessary to be involved in a court case. The classic cases are rape cases, whereby the trauma is often replicated and exacerbated by the court case. One hears of women who say they were raped twice, 'Once in the incident and then in court.' This is too simplistic a view as it ignores some of the other traumatic experiences that any rape victim might experience: the original incident, any prior incidents triggered by it, the trauma, stresses or indignities suffered while undergoing medical and police investigation, explanations and consequences to any partnership, explanations and consequences to friends and family, the court case, and any media exposure. TIR can be employed in addressing any and all of the above insofar as they can be compartmentalized. Often an initiating incident (such as a rape) will not reach a point of resolution while environmental factors seem to keep it an issue in the present. In such cases counsellors would obviously need to use any and all of their other supportive skills to enable the client to get through the entire experience.

2. Unfinished Business

Traumas can either trigger unfulfilled intentions or create them. A sudden death often creates feelings of guilt or regret, things we wished we had said or done and didn't, things we said or did we wished we hadn't and never apologized for. Any trauma, by its nature, interrupts our plans. It is unexpected. It cuts across our schemas for living. It leaves us with things unsaid and undone.

The witnessing of a trauma – for example, the Dunblane massacre – can be traumatic in itself or can trigger past incidents – bereavements in our own lives or in others. Things we should have said and done, graves we should have visited and did not, relatives that should have been contacted and were not.

Relationships can be formed at the time of a trauma by virtue of a mutual experience: for example, two people injured in a train crash exchange phone numbers but never get together again. The intention was formed but not fulfilled. Attention remains on the incident and helps keep it present instead of past. When unfulfilled intentions can be identified by a client in a counselling session they can be explored to the point of recognition and deciding to fulfil them or deciding not to fulfil them. Either way, the attention on them can be dispersed and the issue settled.

For example, a train driver who suffered when a person committed suicide by throwing himself in front of the train remained stuck with questions about who the person was and why he had committed suicide. Pondering this question, this driver (inadvertently) created a 'cognitive loop'. The unanswered questions meant that the incident was kept alive and in the present. His constant posing of the question in his own mental environment (which did not contain the answer) can be seen as a source of continual triggering of the trauma. The solution in this case was for the counsellor to identify the question and have the client actually provide himself with the answers that were available in incident records. In this case, the 'unfinished business' was easily finished. That is not always the case, but where traumatic incidents raise questions that can be dealt with by references to records, witnesses, video tapes, etc., then this should obviously be done.

Intentions highlighted or created by a trauma that have no practical solution are more difficult to deal with, especially in the case of bereavement. The whole phenomenon of regret, the mental effort to rearrange the past, comes into play, with the effect that this again tends to keep a trauma in the present rather than the past. Identifying the unfinished business seems to be quite beneficial, especially when the client also sees how this contributes to his condition.

Much more difficult to deal with can be the existential type of questions that can be raised by a traumatic experience. 'Why did this happen to me?' 'What did I do to deserve this?' 'What is life (or God) trying to teach me?' Such questions again create a cognitive loop, and while the client ponders them he is constantly referring to information contained in the trauma which perforce keeps it in the present rather than allowing it to become a past experience. Such questions are almost inevitable. A trauma, by definition, is an experience for which a person has no schemata to accommodate. When life and limb have been threatened or destroyed and there is an absence of an explanatory structure, then this may be the key aspect of the trauma that requires resolution.

Such questions, philosophic in nature, are obviously not something a counsellor can supply answers to, nor can he refer the client to where the definitive answers might be found. Yet a client might be very 'hung up' on them. For example, one client experienced a series of assaults. He had coped with them by changing what he did, where he went and a number of attitudes he felt he was displaying. He developed Post-Traumatic Stress Disorder as a result of the last assault. Counselling revealed that the development of the condition was not just a result of accumulated charge but the questions he had formulated as a consequence of similar experiences. 'What is someone trying to tell me?' 'What am I doing wrong?' 'What do I need to change so that this doesn't happen to me again?'

The counsellor's problem when faced with these issues could be: (a) there are no definite answers; (b) there are no referrals possible that might answer the questions; (c) the life-changing event may well require some time for assimilation and accommodation of either the questions or possible answers.

The trauma presents a person with confusion. A client is looking for answers, stability and certainty from the counsellor. Whereas the counsellor can provide the client with understanding of how the trauma might have effected him and enable him to process the experience, the questions arising from it may well be beyond the ken of counsellor and client. In longer term therapy, such existential questions can be explored. In the short term, our experience has been that the *identification* of the issues is of considerable benefit. The client's confusion seems to be lessened or obviscated if the questions raised can be exactly identified and seen in the context of previous experience. In other words, it does not seem to matter so much that a question is not answered as long as the question itself is identified, along with how the question was raised in the first place.

3. Secondary Gain Issues

Where clients have some kind of vested interest in remaining in their traumatized condition this will keep the trauma triggered. This is covered in the next chapter.

In Chapter 8, we cover questions to investigate the points raised in this section.

DESCRIPTION OF THE TWO CASES THAT WILL RUN THROUGHOUT THIS BOOK

Case 1: Mary

Mary was a white 30-year-old married female who was referred for TIR by a colleague who knew that she was suffering with PTSD, having been sexually abused as a child and also suffered an assault by a client. She was a practising counsellor at the time she requested TIR. She said that she had already undertaken a considerable amount of therapy which had helped with a variety of symptoms, but that she still had PTSD.

Psychometric testing confirmed a diagnosis of PTSD. She was given the PENN Inventory (Hammarberg, 1990 – a test for PTSD), the Impact of Event Scale (Horowitz, Wilner & Alvarez, 1979 – a test for PTSD) and a PTSD symptom checklist (Bisbey, 1995). Her score on the PENN Inventory was 29. The PENN Inventory has a cut-off score for a diagnosis of PTSD; a score of 35 or above is considered to be a positive diagnosis while a score above 15 is considered to be symptomatic. Her score on the Impact of Event Scale was 57. This test does not have a cut-off score; however, generally any score over 20 is considered to be indicative of a traumatized person. On the symptom checklist, she indicated she was experiencing the following symptoms.

Intrusion symptoms (one needed to meet Criterion B in the PTSD diagnosis):

- intrusive thoughts of the trauma
- nightmares relating to the trauma
- flashbacks
- strong emotional reactions to sights, sounds or smells associated with the trauma
- strong emotional reactions on anniversaries of the trauma.

Avoidance symptoms (three needed to meet Criterion C in the PTSD diagnosis):

- difficulty watching television programmes pertaining to the trauma
- attempts to avoid thinking about the trauma

- attempts to avoid anything that brings back memories of the trauma
- difficulty or inability to remember important parts of the trauma
- loss of, or lack of, sexual desire or interest.

Arousal symptoms (two needed to meet Criterion D in the PTSD diagnosis):

- difficulty falling or staying asleep
- feeling irritable often or experiencing outbursts of anger
- being consistently very aware of everything going on around you
- startling easily.

Mary's diagnosis of PTSD was confirmed during an interview. She was then educated about TIR and a history session was scheduled. We will be following Mary's case throughout the book and verbatim examples of her sessions are included in most chapters.

Case 2: Renee

Renee was a white 46-year-old married female presenting herself for trauma counselling having been shot in the back by her alcoholic husband some four months earlier. She still had numerous 12-gauge shotgun pellets in her body that she had been advised would 'work their way out' rather than the alternative of undergoing surgery which would create further scarring. Her husband, Roger, was in jail charged with attempted murder and awaiting trial.

Having been in hospital for a week, Renee was off work and taking anti-depressant medication. Psychometric tests, including a PTSD symptom checklist, the PENN Inventory (Hammarberg, 1990) and the Impact of Event Scale (Horowitz, Wilner & Alvarez, 1979) showed her symptoms to be consistent with the DSM IV diagnosis of PTSD. She was sleeping only four or five hours per night, generally anxious, afraid of leaving her home, prone to uncontrollable bursts of weeping, and any loud noises or 'rows' would give rise to feelings of terror. The general anxiety varied with days of depression, feeling guilty, and 'angry at everyone'. She had recently initiated divorce proceedings and was filling her time 'moping around the house' and coping with her two children, both of whom were heroin addicts. Her score on the PENN Inventory was 49. Her score on the Impact of Event Scale was 53. On the symptom checklist she indicated that she was experiencing the following symptoms.

Intrusion symptoms (one needed to meet Criterion B in the PTSD diagnosis):

- intrusive thoughts relating to the crime
- nightmares relating to the crime
- flashbacks
- strong emotional reactions when reminded of the crime.

Avoidance symptoms (three needed to meet Criterion C in the PTSD diagnosis):

- difficulty reading anything about crime or crime victims
- difficulty watching television relating to crime or crime victims
- lowered interest in usually enjoyed activities
- feeling as though things that are happening are not real – or detached from your thoughts, feelings and possibly your body
- loss of, or lack of, sexual desire or interest
- feeling detached and separate from others.

Arousal symptoms (two needed to meet Criterion D in the PTSD diagnosis):

- difficulty falling or staying asleep
- feeling irritable or experiencing outbursts of anger
- startling easily.

After the initial session establishing the general picture, explaining her support systems and educating her in trauma counselling (she had no previous experience of any kind of psychotherapy or counselling), a history-taking session was planned. We will be following Renee's case throughout the book and verbatim samples of her sessions are used as examples in each chapter.

3

WHO IS SUITABLE?

In Chapter 2 we focused on the broader picture of PTSD and some of the theory that underpins the use of Traumatic Incident Reduction. In this chapter we return to specific issues relating to the choice of TIR as the specific treatment for a client. We cover when it is suitable to use TIR as the primary counselling method and when TIR can be integrated into a treatment plan as well as when it is not suitable to use this method.

WHEN THIS METHOD OF WORKING IS NOT APPROPRIATE

As in any other profession, different tools are needed to do different jobs. For example, let us say that someone wants to hang a picture on the wall. She has a choice in the way she goes about doing this task. She can place the picture on the wall by hanging it on a hook which is connected to the wall with a nail. She can use a hook which is connected to the wall with a screw. She can use the nail only. She can use the screw only. She could even take double-stick tape and put the picture on the wall using that. Screwdrivers don't work for nails. Hammers don't work for screws. Double-stick tape doesn't hold much weight. If she chooses to use the double-stick tape, it is likely that the picture may stay on the wall for a short while but will eventually fall off the wall and may even break when it does.

She is limited by the number and variety of tools she has and the ways in which she knows how to use these tools. She is also limited by the condition of the wall and what might be inside it. Sometimes the wall turns out to be made of plasterboard which crumbles easily and sometimes there are pipes or electrical cables behind the wall which would be disastrous to cut or break.

If a person is not sure of the proper way to use either a hammer or a screwdriver, she may well have to learn by asking someone else to teach her. She could learn by reading a book about hanging pictures, but this may not give her a full understanding. It would certainly be better than nothing and would likely produce a result that somewhat resembles the ideal, but it may not produce the ideal result.

This analogy carries into psychotherapy and counselling although the strengths and weaknesses of a method are not usually as clear cut as they are when deciding on hanging a picture on the wall. There are a variety of ways in which a counsellor can work with a client who is traumatized. All of the ways have their strengths and weaknesses and all work better in some circumstances than in others. All counsellors working in this area should be aware of the tools available, their limitations and their strengths, if not having more than one tool themselves. A tool or 'technique' as would be appropriate in counselling is merely a method or vehicle that enables the client to *access and process* the material (in this case a trauma) being addressed to a point of resolution.

The first key to choosing the right tool is properly recognizing the task that is facing the counsellor. This is a matter of diagnosis and will not be fully addressed here as it is a separate subject requiring considerable space and depth that goes beyond the scope of this book. The second is knowing the strengths and limitations of the various tools. Some of this is covered in Appendix 1 with an overview of the methods currently available. The rest is covered here by looking at the specific strengths and limitations of Traumatic Incident Reduction and related methods of working.

There are a variety of limitations to TIR and related methods and each one will be discussed in turn. The first of the limitations is use of TIR in cases where the client is not adequately motivated. All forms of counselling require adequate motivation on the part of the client in order to be successful. This is not because of a placebo effect or any non-specific therapist effect. This is simply because most forms of counselling require a lot of hard and possibly painful work on the part of the client, so if there is not sufficient motivation to stick with the treatment, it obviously will not succeed.

This is particularly true with Traumatic Incident Reduction as the exposure part of the work can be very intense and the client needs to be motivated in order to complete the work in session. Clients who are not motivated or motivated for reasons other than to get better will not be successful when using this method. TIR requires the client to feel safe enough and confident enough to tell the counsellor whatever comes to his mind regardless of relevance. This can only happen when the client is motivated to change.

There are a variety of reasons for a client being unmotivated. Sometimes clients are aware that they are unmotivated internally – for example, when attending therapy because of external pressure because a spouse has threatened divorce if they do not attend or a court has ordered therapy. Other times clients are not aware that they are unmotivated to get better. These reasons, on a less conscious level, are often referred to as 'secondary gain issues'. Secondary gain refers to the benefits (conscious or unconscious) of having the particular condition (such as a diagnosis of Post-Traumatic Stress Disorder).

For example, the symptoms of PTSD may well be very aversive but a benefit of having these symptoms may well be that someone does not have to work every day and instead is able to pursue a course of study he wished to pursue but never had the time. Should this person get better, then he may no longer be financially able to pursue the course of study but may have to return to work. This issue would have to be addressed as soon as it came to light (preferably at the outset of the work) or the person may well not get better because the consequences of getting better outweigh the benefits.

If the client is currently receiving disability payments or if she has litigation for damages pending then the consequences of getting better might mean a great financial loss. If the client feels (on any level – conscious or unconscious) that the resolution of the condition will leave her worse off then she is unlikely to get better. When these issues are not addressed, the person is unlikely to improve no matter what method of treatment is employed.

The second limitation involves psychotropic medication or psychoactive substance use. Many psychotropic medications or psychoactive substances cloud awareness (usually through some type of sedative effect). TIR requires the person to use as much of his awareness and attention as possible in the session. By definition, available awareness and attention is reduced by virtue of the unresolved traumatic incidents. In addition, sleep disturbance is one of the most common symptoms of unresolved traumatic incidents and this too lowers the amount of available awareness and attention. Therefore, adding to this any further clouding of awareness (through the use of some psychoactive medications and/or alcohol or non-prescribed drugs) makes the task even more difficult and, in some cases, impossible. This causes a problem inasmuch as quite frequently psychotropic medication is prescribed either for co-morbid depression or for sleep disturbance, and when medication is not prescribed many people resort to increased use of alcohol and non-prescribed sedatives for the same reason.

Regarding the issue of prescribed medication, TIR does not work well in situations where the client is taking a major tranquillizer or neuroleptic (such as Haloperidol, Stellazine and the like). In these situations, TIR would not be the treatment of choice. (Most conditions which require the use of such major tranquillizers are contraindications in and of themselves.)

The ability to engage in TIR is also negatively affected by certain anti-depressant medications. The ones that have the strongest negative effect are those that have a sedative effect. This refers primarily to such medications as tricyclic anti-depressants (imipramine, amitripytiline, desipramine, Dothiepin). All of these have a sedative effect and are often prescribed because a client is having a sleep disturbance. Lack of sleep (e.g. 2–3 hours per night or sleep that results in the client feeling exhausted when he turns up for his session) has a worse effect than the sedative contained in the anti-depressants. So if the client cannot get a reasonable amount of sleep (and come to session with a reasonable amount of energy) if he does not take the medication, then it is better that he takes the medication. The counsellor can arrange sessions for the part of the day in which the client has the most energy. **We are not suggesting that the counsellor tell the client to stop taking his medication. This should not be done without consultation with his general practitioner or psychiatrist.** We are suggesting that in cases where the sedative type anti-depressant is not absolutely necessary, the client consider discussing stopping the medication with his general practitioner as treatment will be more effective without the medication.

The ability to engage in TIR does not seem to be affected by the new generation of anti-depressants, SSRIs (such as Prozac and Seroxat), as these seem to have much less of a sedative effect. Often we find that a client has developed depression AFTER developing PTSD. When this is the case, treating the PTSD often resolves the depression (Bisbey, 1995). In these situations, we prefer if the client is not on anti-depressant medication of any type. As long as the client (a) is not actively suicidal and (b) has enough energy to engage in the treatment, we much prefer that he be medication free.

The ability to engage in TIR is affected by anti-anxiety medications (minor tranquillizers) such as Valium (Diazepam), Xanax and Librium. Again, this tends to cloud awareness (particularly in relation to experiencing emotions) and it is preferable that the client not be on this type of medication if the counsellor is intending to use TIR. For those clients who are experiencing panic attacks, medications such as propanalol (beta blockers) do not seem to have the same negative effect despite the fact that they shut off the physical symptoms of stress and anxiety. Again, if at all possible, we prefer clients to be medication free.

In cases where clients are prescribed Lithium for bipolar disorder (manic depression), we have found that TIR is not effective if the client does NOT take his medication. When the client does take his medication, TIR has seemed to work extremely well. This is because when a client is experiencing mania or manic symptoms it is often difficult for him to follow one train of thought to its conclusion; consequently he ends up looking at all incidents and issues as connected. When the client is taking Lithium, it becomes possible for him to focus his attention and therefore TIR works well in allowing him to examine one issue at a time.

The same issues as arise with sedatives containing anti-depressant medication arise with sedatives or barbiturates (sleep medications such as Temazapam) and the same rules should be applied. Opiates also cause the same clouding of awareness and have two effects that cause problems in this situation. The first is that opiates (particularly Zydol) tend to make flashbacks, any associated hallucinations and nightmares more intense and more frequent. The second is that they cloud awareness, so using TIR to work through the actual traumatic incidents becomes extremely difficult and, in some cases, impossible. This is a particular problem in the case of dependence, where physical injuries require the use of opiate pain killers (particularly Zydol) on a regular basis. We request that clients refrain from the use of headache remedies containing codeine within 24 hours of a session (with long-term use usually at least 48 hours is necessary). In cases where the pain is continual, another method of working may need to be found.

Alcohol consumption is a problem for the same reasons. We request that clients refrain from the use of alcohol the day before a session. Clients who cannot comply with this request are not treated with TIR. The two most common co-diagnoses occurring with Post-Traumatic Stress Disorder are depression and substance abuse/dependence. Self-medication with alcohol is a common phenomenon in clients who have PTSD. If a client cannot comply with the rules around alcohol consumption, we usually refer for another form of treatment. In the case of a diagnosis of substance abuse/dependence, we refer the client for treatment for these issues first and then will accept the client for trauma treatment.

WHAT HAPPENS WHEN THESE RULES ARE NOT FOLLOWED?

What might happen if a client is 'drugged' in some way is that she gets into the middle of the incident and cannot find her way out of it. The levels of anxiety and other negative emotions increase and her thinking is not clear enough to make the connections and associations that allow the cognitive shift to take place. Consequently, the client gets 'stuck' and the session ends poorly. This is not always the case but it has happened often enough for these rules to be put in place. If in doubt, check with a TIR supervisor about the particular case or choose to work with another method (such as one that focuses on symptom management). Keep in mind that these rules do not have ANY moral judgement attached to them – they are simply born out of experience with the strengths and limitations of this technique.

WHAT ABOUT THE THERAPIST/COUNSELLOR?

In our experience, TIR requires just as much energy and attention for the counsellor as it does for the client; therefore, it is best if the counsellor follows the same rules as the client if at all possible when it comes to ingestion of psychoactive substances or any kind of psychotropic medication. These are the rules that are given to students on the TIR training workshop and invariably, when someone does not follow these rules, it becomes obvious in the training session the next day. We repeat: this is not a MORAL issue. It has nothing to do with the relative benefits or negative effects of the use of alcohol or other drugs. It has everything to do with the counsellor's ability to stay in contact with the client during the session and take the session to its desired conclusion. Different people are affected to different degrees by psychoactive substances. The rule of thumb is that if there is a possible negative effect the following day, it is best to abstain entirely. We realize that a lot of counsellors ignore this rule of thumb periodically. Habitually, this can cause the counsellor to be considerably less effective and does a disservice to the client.

OTHER DIAGNOSES

TIR is not useful in cases where a client has a psychotic disorder. This appears to be for some of the same reasons stated above for substance dependence or psychoactive medication. The client needs as much awareness and attention that can possibly be focused in order to work through the traumatic incidents. In psychotic disorders, clients often cannot focus long enough on a particular train of thought to fully process the information to a logical conclusion. In these cases, the psychotic disorder must be treated first and then the traumatic material addressed. There are many more appropriate methods to use in working with people who have these conditions.*

TIR is not terribly effective in cases where the client has a severe personality disorder. The rule of thumb is that if a counsellor would not normally treat clients who have severe personality disorders (such as borderline personality disorder) without TIR or related methods, then she should not attempt to treat them with these methods. If a counsellor does not use a system of diagnosis which includes these categories, here are some warning signs that TIR might not be the treatment of choice. (**Please note: these are warning signs only. They do not indicate that a diagnosis of personality disorder should be made. One warning sign is not enough to contraindicate using TIR. When there are multiple warning signs, TIR is likely to be contraindicated. If in doubt, seek supervision.**)

1. The client has been to multiple therapists to attempt to handle the traumatic material and none of these has worked. **In addition**, the client has little or nothing positive to say about his work with these therapists.
2. The client has unrealistic positive expectations of the counsellor's ability to treat him.
3. The client has numerous reasons why he cannot do as the counsellor suggests (such as get a good night's sleep) or answers any suggestion with 'Yes, but . . .'.
4. The client has a long history of chaotic relationships with little evidence of any type of stable positive relationship.
5. The client has a history of repeatedly engaging in self-destructive behaviour such as self-mutilation or suicide attempts.

If these signs are present, it is recommended that TIR is not used as the treatment of choice or that considerable preparatory work is done (in establishing a stable relationship with the client) before TIR is attempted and supervision received from a more experienced TIR practitioner who also has experience working with this client group.†

---

* Psychotropic medication is usually necessary before clients who have psychotic disorders benefit from 'talk' therapies. In some cases, experienced practitioners can integrate some of the TIR method and philosophy into their treatment of traumatized clients who have psychotic disorders. However, this is the exception rather than the rule.

† Transference is often a problem when attempting to use TIR with clients who have a personality disorder. We have developed a method of addressing transference so that it does not intrude into the TIR sessions. This is discussed in our next book.

The counsellor will not be able to use TIR immediately if the person has an active problem that is taking up her attention. There are a variety of related interventions that can be used in this situation. Unblocking is covered in depth in Chapter 6. In these situations, the counsellor must deal with the person's immediate problem before he can use TIR.

The last time when the counsellor may not be able to use TIR is if the trauma is still continuing. In these cases it is possible that the client may be unable to examine the effects of the trauma because she doesn't see an end to it. For example, if someone is in a situation in which domestic violence is happening on a regular basis, she may not be able to use TIR to examine the trauma as she feels it unsafe to do so. In these situations, the person's safety must be established before TIR will be useful. This is by no means a black and white issue, however; in many cases of domestic violence, clients have been able to use TIR to examine past incidents while still living in the violent environment, and in fact this has been what has led to their being able finally to leave the situation.

OPTIMUM CONDITIONS ON A SESSION TO SESSION BASIS

As mentioned above, an adequate amount of sleep is necessary in order for TIR to be successful. This appears to be for two reasons: one is the amount of free awareness and attention the person has to focus on the incident and move through it to a successful conclusion; the second is the actual physical energy necessary to confront painful material until a point of resolution is reached.

In cases where sleep disturbance is a significant problem there are a variety of ways to work around this. One is to schedule sessions for the time of day when the person is most alert and most energetic. The second is to provide facilities for the person to take a short nap prior to any session if at all possible. The third is to refer the person to the general practitioner for sleep medication and to schedule sessions for later in the day when the sedative effects of the medication have worn off.

In addition, an adequate amount of food is necessary in order for TIR to be successful. This is true for the same reasons – it is difficult for a person to focus when he is hungry and the food provides energy to get through the session. We recommend that our clients eat a small meal or a snack prior to session.

This can be a problem in cases of eating disorders. When a client has anorexia, she often does not have the physical energy to sustain this type of work. In fact, there is one psychiatrist who believes that clients who weigh under 5 stone do not have the energy to think properly at all and so therapies that involve introspection and talking will not work in these cases. TIR can only be done in these situations when the client actually eats immediately prior to the session. Even then, less frequent and shorter sessions are more productive.

When a client has bulimia, TIR is most effective just after the client has eaten AND kept the food down. If the client is of normal bodyweight despite the bulimia (e.g. she does not also have anorexia), TIR can be effective in handling traumatic incidents.

When considering ME or chronic fatigue syndrome; energy is one of the primary problems for ME sufferers. In order to do TIR one needs energy. By definition, this makes it difficult to use TIR with ME sufferers. It is not impossible to do, but counsellors must bear in mind the energy consequences of the session itself. TIR should be scheduled for when the client is at her best in terms of energy, and sessions should not be done intensively. The client should expect to need some recovery time (sometimes stretching into a few days) following the session and not automatically see this as a setback. The client should be prepared to be more tired rather than less tired initially during a course of TIR. When these conditions are followed, TIR can be quite effective in helping people who have ME to resolve past trauma.

We recommend that thorough history-taking and assessment are done prior to beginning TIR with any client. We find that this process:

- helps to engage the client and establish necessary therapeutic alliance
- helps the client to put some of the trauma into context with the rest of her life
- allows the therapist to identify clients who will not benefit from this method of working in the beginning stages of treatment
- allows the therapist to consider avenues of referral when TIR is not an appropriate treatment choice
- allows the therapist to work with a supervisor in planning how to address the variety of issues using TIR and other related techniques
- allows the therapist to gain the advice of a supervisor in deciding whether TIR is the treatment of choice now – or possibly in the future.

Quite often, it is possible to use TIR within a few sessions of beginning work with a client. However, sometimes it is necessary to use other clinical skills (either related methods or another method of working) in order to create an optimum environment in which TIR can be used successfully. Having a thorough assessment period allows the counsellor to make these decisions accurately and do the most effective thing for that client at that particular time. It saves time in the long run and prevents having to 'fly by the seat of your pants'. It allows the counsellor to develop a reasonable treatment plan and to inform the client of the rationale behind the way in which they are working. Often the difference between keeping a client engaged in the work and losing the client is the degree to which the counsellor is able to choose the appropriate intervention at the appropriate time. It is almost impossible to do this if the counsellor does not have some type of assessment period. Even with intense exposure-based treatments, drop out is much lower if the client is adequately prepared, and in order to adequately prepare the client the counsellor must know something about him (above and beyond the presenting problem). These issues are less of a concern in a peer counselling setting where the client's expectations tend to be somewhat less stringent. In a professional counselling setting, these issues are crucial.

The final reason for doing a full assessment and history-taking is highlighting areas of interest to examine. It is our experience that often the particular incident with which the client comes to therapy is not the only incident that has impacted upon him and caused the development of symptoms. Many times this incident turns out to be insignificant in comparison with other things examined in the counselling. If the counsellor does a full assessment, then she is able to offer the client a choice of what to address, which tends to make for more thorough and effective treatment. It is the difference between treating the symptoms and treating the underlying problems. In the following chapter, we outline further our rationale for a thorough assessment process and provide guidelines for using our methods of assessment as the first stage in a client's counselling programme.

4

ENGAGING THE CLIENT

We have examined the theoretical constructs behind TIR, the preparations for using TIR including the clients with whom this method will be most helpful, and now we move on to the actual treatment process. In this chapter we cover our method of assessment and history-gathering and our method of educating clients in relation to TIR and the counselling process. We discussed some client education in Chapter 2 when we examined information-processing models of trauma. We hope that counsellors will be able to integrate the two methods of education (TIR specific and information-processing models) and develop their own style that they can adapt to suit the individual client.

TRANSCRIPTS

In this chapter we introduce some excerpts from session transcripts of the two clients whom we are following throughout the book. Transcripts, by their nature, are quite sterile and dry and do not really present an adequate picture of the session as they do not include all of the non-verbal communication that occurs during the session. It is often the non-verbal communication that establishes the connection between counsellor and client – the counsellor's reaction to what the client discloses in the session. Appropriate non-verbal and verbal communication are essential to engage a client in the therapeutic process. We educate clients as to the purpose of a thorough assessment and history so that they are fully prepared for the number of questions we will ask and the personal nature of these questions. One of the transcripts includes a sample of this education prior to beginning the Counselling Assessment Form. In order to make the transcript excerpts more realistic, we have included some notes relating to non-verbal communication which were taken at the time of the sessions. However, even with these notes, the full flavour of the session may be hard to grasp.

ASSESSMENT AND HISTORY-TAKING: USING THE COUNSELLING ASSESSMENT FORM

TIR is often used with traumatized clients by practitioners with no previous knowledge of the client. In these circumstances, thorough familiarization with the client's present disposition and history is preferable (although not always immediately possible, as will be noted later). After establishing the client's presenting problem (a description of what they think their condition is and why they are seeking counselling), the first step in the treatment plan would normally be taking a thorough history. 'The Counselling Assessment Form' (reprinted in full in Appendix 1) is an example of what we use.

As mentioned in the previous chapter, a thorough history-taking using the Counselling Assessment Form fulfils several functions.

1. Establishing the context of the *individual's trauma*. The current codification of Post-Traumatic Stress Disorder, categorizations of types of trauma such as individual crime victim classifications (e.g. rape, mugging, etc.) and the debriefing approach tend to highlight the similarities of people's experience and ignore the differences. Obviously trauma is not just a social construction. For the individual, it is a unique experience that occurred in the unique context of their own bodies, minds, personal and social environments, each of which have the potential to either maintain the traumatized state or aid recovery. The Counselling Assessment Form is calculated to focus on the individual and establish the personal context in which their trauma has become embedded.

Evidence that the trauma has become embedded is that the client has a diagnosis of PTSD as opposed to ASD (Acute Stress Disorder). A person could conceptualize the client's inability to recover as the trauma having 'networked' in interaction with the client's past experiences, their body, mental constructs and social situation. In effect, it has 'taken root'. Efforts to help trauma victims with education relating to PTSD and group debriefings may prevent a trauma taking root or aid recovery. If recovery has not occurred, then the client's *individual* context has become part of the trauma and its resolution depends on addressing it from that perspective.

2. Gathering diagnostic information. Without a full client history it is difficult to establish a firm diagnosis of PTSD and difficult to establish the existence or non-existence of other co-diagnoses with implications for treatment. The history enables other syndromes to be identified which, together with psychometric tests, provide a reasonable background on which treatment planning can be based.

3. **Building a therapeutic alliance**.   While the identification of PTSD, the similarities between people's experiences and symptoms and the normalization of them has some therapeutic value, clients can also see categorizations as devaluing their own unique situation. The intense interest the counsellor takes in the client's full life experience during the assessment helps to redress the balance. Trauma techniques, including TIR, could be seen as quite mechanical and impersonal, but the application of this 'system' should be as a structure that facilitates and empowers the client to access, 'process' (assimilate and accommodate) the qualia of her own experience.* The attitude of the counsellor during the history session(s) is most important. The counsellor is there to listen, learn and acknowledge the client, not to comment or interpret. This is the opportunity for the client to feel safe in talking about himself without having to go into the intimate detail of painful events or subjects. It is the opportunity for the counsellor to become familiarized with the client's world view and the major players within it. Later on, when TIR is targeted on specific events, it saves the client long explanations of the context, key identities, places and activities.

The recognition of the present and historical context also allows the client to broaden his attention from where it might be immediately focused (or fixated) and begin to see where it is rooted. While the counsellor may observe the client making such connections, it is not actively promoted. The character of the client's trauma network, what and where it was rooted, is the desired outcome that naturally follows detailed inspection of perhaps many individual incidents. The establishment of patterns and connections is not something that should be pre-empted by an 'informed counsellor' or decided upon in advance by a client hungry for answers and explanations.

WHEN THOROUGH HISTORY-GATHERING IS NOT POSSIBLE

There are some occasions where it is not possible or desirable to engage in a full history-gathering and assessment before actually doing something active to aid the client. It may be clear from the outset that the client's attention is flooded with a trauma and requiring him to complete psychometric questionnaires or discuss his past history would not only be

---

* Qualia is defined as 'The simple, uninterpreted elements of experience' (Reber, 1985, p. 627), or: What clients can contact in their mental environment before they have made sense of it. This could include images, emotions, thoughts or any perception.

beyond his capacity but if attempted, might traumatize him further. In such instances, the counsellor would have to use his own judgement as to an appropriate response which might include anything from the normalizing and grounding activities, such as providing a cup of tea and just listening, to medical intervention.

In the case of a client who is not distressed to the point where grounding techniques or medical intervention is needed, then TIR can be employed straight away to enable the client to discharge the immediate material their attention is on. In this case, a counsellor would not expect a full 'end point' having used the procedure, but would be satisfied with an alleviation of current distress, 'feeling better about it' and the client's return of control over his attention. When the latter is established, or in a later session, it should be possible to do the history-gathering.

History-taking itself has the liability of triggering past events or present problematical situations without doing anything about them. It is for this reason that counsellors should not go into any more detail than necessary when using a history-gathering questionnaire. For example, if the counsellor asked 'Have you experienced any incidents of domestic violence?' and the client said 'Yes, I was sexually abused', he might ask 'When?' or 'Over what period of time?', note the answer down and move on. The counsellor would not ask what happened or even by whom unless it was volunteered, and even then he would not allow much space for the client to go into details. The history-gathering process provides a structure which enables the client to compartmentalize and contain those painful experiences and situations as distinct from other happier or non-problematical ones with a view to selectively addressing them in turn, gradually, and in a manner which minimizes the client's discomfort.

However, it is possible that during the history session(s) the client becomes triggered into a trauma which is so distressing that he loses the capacity to direct his own attention, making it impossible to continue with the history. In this instance, TIR can be used immediately to discharge the incident. (See also the section on band aids in Chapter 9.) Experience has shown that this is a rare occurrence, but it sometimes happens – most usually in cases in which the counsellor does not adequately control the communication in the session.

More rarely a client with low ego strength or in a highly sensitive state cannot be asked anything without triggering distressing issues. In this case an entirely different intervention will be needed. In this type of situation, a referral to a supervisor is advised so that further diagnostic investigation can be completed and an appropriate referral for treatment can be sought. Where possible in such situations, in addition to a Counselling Assessment

Form, the supervisor will often use psychometric testing and ask additional interview questions to determine a possible diagnosis.

The Counselling Assessment Form is normally completed in one session of 1 to 2 hours. Occasionally it may take longer – up to three sessions. Clients should be informed of its purpose to begin with and generally they find it a therapeutic activity in itself.

EXAMPLES FROM THE TWO CASES: THE COUNSELLING ASSESSMENT FORM

Below are excerpts from the Counselling Assessment Forms from the two clients whose cases we are following throughout the book. Follow-up questions that are not part of the standard Counselling Assessment Form are in **bold**. Follow-up questions are asked whenever the counsellor feels more information is needed, either for his understanding or for diagnostic purposes. In these examples, the client's responses are in *italics*. The counsellor's questions are in regular print and observations are in brackets in regular print.

Case 1: Mary

This was done in one session which took 90 minutes.

(The counsellor's tone of voice throughout the session is gentle and reassuring. Despite the fact that the acknowledgements look sharp or brusque in print, the client reports that they come across as 'caring and safe'. This is communicated through tone of voice, use of appropriate eye contact and use of appropriate gestures – such as the counsellor nodding her head to encourage the client, and a relaxed body posture on the part of the counsellor.)

As we discussed earlier, the more information I have about your life, the easier it will be for me to help you. What I typically do is over a session or two, ask my clients a long list of questions that explore their lives, past and present, and touch on future goals. These include some questions about symptoms but mostly focus on your life experience. (Mary is nodding during this description.) I won't ask you to go into a great deal of detail about any area – just to give me enough information so that I can create a treatment plan; however, some of the questions I will ask you are quite personal. Does this sound OK to you?

Yes. It sounds fine. Are we going to be dealing with issues as they come up?

No. What I usually do is get an overview and then create a treatment plan that uses the methods of working I think will be most appropriate given your individual situation. Some clients find the process to be a relief because they have the opportunity to take an overview of their lives, others find it quite painful because a lot of areas are being touched upon without being dealt with in the session. If you find it very painful, we will do some work at the end of the session to help you feel somewhat better before you leave. If you want to stop at any time during the session, just let me know. Is this OK with you?

Yes. It sounds fine.

OK. We'll get started then. Are you upset or cross with anyone or anything at this time?

With my mother and with my supervisor. (Mary is fidgeting in the chair. No follow-up question is asked as the counsellor was already aware of the situations that led to these upsets.)

OK. Do you feel threatened by anything or anyone at this time?

No. One of my client's husband's has made threats but there is no real danger.

OK. Have you received previous counselling?

Yes. From ages 11–14 I saw a school counsellor. Don't remember much about those sessions. For the past six years have been in therapy weekly. Now I only go once a fortnight. Prior to that, I saw someone in college for a while. I saw someone about nine years ago but only for a few sessions. I had one session of rebirthing – but it was disastrous (very charged – Mary speaking in a very angry tone). *I was in group therapy for a few years. I also did some couples work with my husband.*

All right. What benefits did you have from counselling?

From the past six years, lots. Counsellor was very supportive. I was able to trust her and changed lots of behaviour, thoughts and feelings. Lots of issues resolved. The group work was good – helped with interpersonal issues. (Mary is smiling and sitting in a relaxed manner while she talks about this area.)

Fine. Is there anything you expected to achieve in counselling and didn't?

Yes. No more PTSD. (Mary smiles and the counsellor smiles as well.)

Got it. Have you had any alternative therapy or treatment?

Yes. The rebirthing session I mentioned and I was involved in a charismatic Christian healing group for a while. They gave support but it wasn't what I was looking for.

OK. Are you currently involved in any alternative therapy or treatment?

No.

(End of transcript.)

Note that the first section of the Counselling Assessment Form deals with current issues – areas on which the client's attention is currently focused – and asks about potential danger. We examine these areas first because, if the client is under threat, he will not be able to concentrate on anything else. The same is true in cases where the client has a current problem (as discussed earlier in the chapter). We may need to deal with these areas prior to finishing the history or as the first step in the counselling programme.

The next section of the form deals with any previous therapy and the outcome of this therapy. We use this section to examine past interventions so that we can avoid things that have not worked for the client in the past and begin to examine the client's counselling goals. In addition, we use this section diagnostically, to help decide if TIR is the appropriate intervention. For example, some clients have had negative experiences with a variety of previous counsellors and methods of counselling. If we are to be successful with these clients, we must make sure that they are not carrying over their expectations from the previous counselling experience. In these cases, we often use Unblocking on previous counselling with the client prior to addressing the trauma issues. This is discussed in depth in Chapter 6.

Below is a second excerpt from Mary's Counselling Assessment Form. This transcript is included to help the reader see the connection between the client's response on the counselling assessment form and the trauma list constructed by the counsellor for use in the TIR sessions.

The next group of questions are relating to your relationship with family members.

What relationship? (Mary laughs.) *Seriously, I'm OK to continue.*

OK. Is your mother living?

Yes.

OK. What is your relationship with your mother?

Appalling. (This appears very charged – Mary's face is red, she has an angry tone to her voice.) *She blames me for not telling her that I was abused which caused her to stay in the relationship. She has no boundaries.*

Got it. Is your father living?

Yes.

What is your relationship with your father?

Non-existent. I haven't seen him since I confronted him about the abuse around Christmas in 1989. (Client's expression is non-descript so the counsellor asks a follow-up question.)

OK. **Was it traumatic when you confronted your father?**

No. It was scary but I was supported by my aunt and uncle. There's lots of stuff around my relationship with my father but nothing around having no relationship with him currently. I'm fine with that. (Mary looks more relaxed.)

All right. Have you any brothers living?

No. Mother had three miscarriages – two of them were boys. I didn't know until I was an adult. (Mary's tone of voice is neutral. She still looks relaxed.)

OK. Have you any sisters living?

Yes. One is two years younger than me – Angela, and the other is ten years younger – Susan, and lives with us.

Fine. What is your relationship like with them?

With Susan – excellent now. I stopped seeing the family seven years ago and initially she felt abandoned but now it is fine. With Angela – no real relationship. (Mary is moving about in the chair when talking about this.)

OK. Have your parents ever been divorced?

No. Mother left father five years ago. She tried to leave three times previously. I found it very traumatic. After the third time she left, he tried to kill me. (This is extremely charged. Mary is visibly upset and begins to cry. She takes a Kleenex from the box on the table. Counsellor's expression is empathic. Counsellor waits quietly until Mary's tears have subsided. Counsellor's tone of voice is more gentle when moving on to the next question.)

(End of transcript excerpt.)

What follows is an excerpt from Renee's Counselling Assessment Form, the second case that we are following throughout this book. The excerpt is taken from the middle of the Counselling Assessment Form.

Case 2: Renee

This was done in three sessions – in part because there was a considerable amount of material and in part because a lot was going on in Renee's life between sessions which needed attention during each session. Her husband was held in custody awaiting trial when the counselling sessions began and the trial occurred within a month of beginning counselling. Some of the session time was used to support Renee through the legal process as she had to give evidence and her husband continued to contact her even after sentencing. The rule of thumb is that when an issue or trauma is continuing in the present and the client's attention is on it, that must be the focus of the initial work. The Counselling Assessment Form took approximately 5 hours. (The counsellor's tone of voice throughout the session is gentle and reassuring. Despite the fact that the acknowledgements look sharp or brusque in print, the client reports that they come across as 'supportive'. This is communicated through tone of voice, use of appropriate eye contact and use of appropriate gestures – such as the counsellor nodding his head to encourage the client, and a relaxed body posture on the part of the counsellor.)

Do you have any children?

Angela is 26 and George is 23. (Renee looks upset as she begins to talk about her children.)

What is your relationship like with them?

Both are heroin addicts. The relationships are very erratic. The usual problems when they were at home – court appearances, etc. Angela has been in and out of detox. (This is very charged – Renee is tearful while talking about it. Counsellor gives Renee a Kleenex.)

OK. Other than with the children you mentioned, have you ever been pregnant?

Yes. I had a child at age 17 that was given up for adoption. Father wouldn't have anything to do with me and mother didn't stick up for me. Because I didn't have anyone supporting me – I put him up for adoption. I wouldn't have been able to cope. I had him for six months and have had no contact since. The biggest trauma in this was that dad didn't want to know. (Very charged, very upset and crying. Counsellor waits and checks that Renee is happy to go on. She says that she is and they continue the session. If the client had not recovered from this upset to the point of being able to move on, then this would have been one of those occasions where the counsellor could immediately have used TIR.)

All right. Have you ever been divorced?

Just the current one I am going through. I have no feelings about it really – I was divorced from him a long time ago is how it feels.

OK. Please tell me about any significant previous romantic relationships you have had.

Chris was my first boyfriend – from age 15½ to 17½. He was the father of the baby I gave up. I was angry with him as I felt used. (Renee is speaking in an angry tone of voice.). *Only other is my husband Roger.*

OK. Have there been any deaths that have affected you?

My father in 1991. Roger's father in 1981. Cousin Alan died 1982. Mother-in-law committed suicide in May 1989. (All of these areas appear charged. Renee is tearful when talking about them and her tone of voice is distressed. In the case of a question eliciting distress, the counsellor allows the client to say what she wants to about it and then moves on.)

(End of transcript excerpt.)

The next transcript excerpt covers the section on drugs and alcohol. For treatment matching and treatment planning, it is very important to know what kind of substances the client is using (if any) and the level of substance use. In this case, the client was very direct in answering the questions. In some cases, clients are wary and answer these questions less than honestly. We recommend that counsellors note any observations that indicate the client might be answering less than honestly. Sometimes it is necessary for the counsellor to go over confidentiality with the client again at this point so that he feels free to answer honestly.

The next group of questions are about medications, drugs and alcohol. All of these areas have a bearing on what methods of counselling will be most helpful to you. That is why I am asking these questions.

That's fine.

Are you currently taking any street drugs?

No.

OK. Have you taken any street drugs in the past?

Used to smoke cigarettes – gave up two years ago.

OK. Do you currently drink alcohol?

Wine when I go out. Don't drink at all when I'm driving. In a pub – couple of drinks.

OK. Have you ever had a different drinking pattern?

Got pissed twice since I split up with Roger – that's all. Not drunk since. Only other time was when I was 15. I've never been a drinker.

OK. Are you taking any prescribed drugs or medicines?

Lofrapamine – anti-depressants. 70 mgs per day.

OK. Have you previously taken any prescribed drugs or medicines?

Amitryptiline anti-depressant years ago. I was on Atavan for depression in 1982. I took them for two years and then stored up some pills and took all of them following an argument with Roger in 1982 in a suicide attempt. I was in hospital in coma and I saw shadowy figures whilst in the coma. I talked to them at the time. After I came out of the coma I got stronger. I was still depressed but much stronger and I didn't take the tablets ever again. It was possibly a near death experience. (Renee's tone of voice indicates that this area is charged.)

(End of transcript excerpt.)

When a client brings up 'near death' or 'paranormal' experiences, the counsellor must remain person-focused and accept what the client is saying. It is crucial that the counsellor shows no shock, worry, or disbelief in his facial expression or tone of voice. These areas are frequently very difficult for a client to talk about and if the counsellor reacts in a negative fashion, the client is unlikely to bring these areas up again. If the client withholds information from the counsellor, this creates problems in the session because the client's attention is usually on the information he is withholding rather than on the area being addressed. In addition, the counsellor may be missing out on information that would help him to know where the client is in the process of the session.

It is clear from Renee's responses regarding drugs and alcohol that these are not problem areas for her. Remember that if someone is actively abusing substances, TIR is not an appropriate treatment method. In this case, we do not have a problem. However, Renee is taking anti-depressants that can have a sedative effect. Because of this, the counsellor decides to schedule sessions for later in the day so Renee will not feel 'hung over' or 'sedated' when she is coming to a session.

While completing the Counselling Assessment Form, the counsellor should at all times be alert for and note emotionally 'charged' areas. The following list comprises the evidence you might find to indicate that a subject area is charged to a greater or lesser degree:

1. Change of skin tone such as sudden paling or flushing of the skin.
2. Affective response (either inappropriate affect – e.g. the client laughs when talking about the death of a parent – or any perceived negative emotion such as anger, fear, or grief or unnatural or nervous laughter).
3. Faltering of communication or a delay in answering that is not followed by an upbeat or positive answer. Reticence to answer. Sudden surge of communication on the subject.
4. Change in eye contact: averting of eye contact or an effort to maintain eye contact.
5. Excessive assertion of no charge or no interest or insignificance of the item.
6. Excessive physical discomfort in the chair, physical movement or expressions that could indicate anxiety or nervousness (such as fiddling with hair). Twitches. Excessive coughing or clearing of the throat.
7. Change of voice tone.
8. Content of the answer indicates that negative emotion is present (such as angry content or highly critical content).
9. Physical indications of embarrassment or statement that the client is embarrassed.
10. Any effort to change the subject.
11. Unwillingness to continue or suddenly wanting a break in the session.
12. Excessive effort to rationalize, explain or justify an answer.
13. Physical pain or discomfort beginning in the session.
14. Agitation or impatience.
15. Interest or mystery – puzzlement, pondering.

Rather than make voluminous notes, counsellors usually use their own system of abbreviations such as the use of stars. One star might indicate mild evidence of charge while four stars might indicate severe charge. This system and the notes are for the counsellor's information and are used only to gain and record the counsellor's observations of the client's responses. At no time should the counsellor decide for the client which of his or her issues are charged or to what degree.

The Counselling Assessment Form constitutes baseline questions to which supplementary questions should be added by the counsellor as needed. A counsellor should always be aware of who is sitting in front of him. An unemployed person will have different stresses than someone who is working. A client's religious education and upbringing may well have produced different attitudes and stresses. When asking supplementary questions, a counsellor should try to avoid stereotyping at the same time. If a Roman Catholic client has had an abortion it does not mean she is now laden with guilt and concerned that she will go to hell. If a counsellor is uncertain about whether an abortion is a charged incident then 'How do you feel about (incident)?' is preferable to 'Did you feel guilty about (incident)?'.

EDUCATING THE CLIENT

Some client education regarding counselling activities is essential at the outset. As we discussed in Chapter 2, this education can include models of trauma and information processing. If a client has no experience of counselling, he can be asked what he expects the counselling to be about and what he expects will happen in the counselling sessions. At this point, any wrong impressions are clarified. For example, some clients think that the counsellor will 'do something' to 'solve' their problems. The counsellor must gently correct this misconception or the client will not be able to properly engage in the counselling process.

We find it useful to tell clients what they can expect in counselling sessions – what we will do, what we expect them to do, and if we are changing what we are doing in the sessions, what the new rules will be. This gives clients more control over the counselling process and helps to establish safety in the sessions.

A client who has had previous counselling should be asked what it consisted of, and without getting too technical, the counsellor should establish what theoretical and practical models were employed in the previous counselling. Differences and similarities between methods are pointed out, any bad experiences with counselling can be explored (often using Unblocking), and positive experiences can be acknowledged. Some of this is done during the counselling assessment session(s), and the rest of this work should be done prior to beginning the actual TIR programme.

Counsellors should be attentive for evidence that a client who has worked extensively and profitably with another therapeutic model has assimilated that model as a grand explanatory theory for their world view. Such a client might experience problems with the TIR method or style of counselling if this were to conflict with the client's earlier education. For example, a client who has received extensive psychoanalysis may, from previous sessions, expect the counsellor to interpret their experience. They might also tend to disregard the impact of later experiences in favour of examining childhood incidents. A client who has received cognitive psychotherapy might believe that the past is relatively unimportant compared to how he thinks about his condition in the present.

Such issues, when present, should come up on the Counselling Assessment Form and a counsellor is advised to be alert for them and educate the client accordingly, being careful not to belittle the client's beliefs. Similarities (there usually are some) between the client's existing understanding and the TIR model can be pointed out and the differences explained to the point where the client feels able to accept them.

It is also possible that clients with no previous experience of counselling enter the process with a belief system that might conflict with the TIR model. For example, a client with strong religious views might have difficulty with the idea of an internal locus of control or personal autonomy. Natural science-oriented clients might have difficulty with the notion that the talking involved in trauma counselling can be beneficial. Our experience is that these issues seldom present a barrier when the client has referred himself for counselling, in which case he is usually open to education and change. It is normally enough to note such issues, discuss them and educate as necessary. *Persuading* the client to drop an existing belief is not recommended, and in the event of the client feeling unable to embrace the TIR model to the point of trying it, they should not be accepted for TIR counselling and another more appropriate method should be found or a referral made that better suits the client's beliefs.

Initial client education includes normalizing their condition, using the principle that trauma symptoms are a normal response to an abnormal experience. We define abnormal as abnormal for *the client*, thus a bereavement can be an abnormal experience and result in trauma symptomatology whether or not the client meets the PTSD diagnostic criteria as per the DSM IV.

We often explain to clients that symptomatology is adaptive – e.g. has helped them to survive. The memories of the trauma are intruding into consciousness as nightmares, flashbacks or intrusive thoughts because the unprocessed material requires conscious processing to restore mental equilibrium and to keep the client in a state of vigilance while the trauma is unresolved. We can posit the idea that PTSD symptomatology is no different from physiological symptomatology – a warning sign that attention is needed to a condition.* If the individual's mental defences, principally repression (comparable with the physiological immune system) were performing adequately, then the incident would be successfully 'parked' to the point where it would not be intruding upon consciousness and causing symptomatology. That there is symptomatology shows that

---

* Refer to the section on Selye and homeostasis in Chapter 2 (p. 20) for more information.

the 'charge' connected with the incident has been sufficient to overwhelm the defences and that this must now be acknowledged, the incident consciously addressed, processed and defences rebuilt.

The normalization process is essential especially where a client with no previous experience of counselling or psychotherapy might think of themselves as a 'patient' or someone with a 'mental disorder'. A person suffering from PTSD, acute stress disorder, or more minor symptoms is not mentally ill. This may need to be emphasized to the client along with the principle that a diagnosis is not the person. The labelling of someone as an 'agoraphobic' is as disempowering as labelling someone as a 'victim'. A more empowering characterization of a client's condition is one that separates the condition from the client – e.g. 'Your symptoms are consistent with *having* a condition known as agoraphobia' or 'Your experience in the train disaster has made you a "victim" with PTSD. We intend to address that experience to the point you recover from it and no longer have to entertain that status.' Diagnosis can be useful as a normalization process and reassuring to the client but becomes a liability if, at the same time, it saddles the client with an identity he feels he cannot change at a time when he is vulnerable to such suggestions.

In general, we point out to clients that PTSD is an *acquired* condition by virtue of an experience (or experiences) and can be differentiated from characterological disorders that might have existed from birth or early development that might be more difficult to address and require long-term psychotherapy. A parallel with physiology can be appropriate in which PTSD could be seen as an acquired infection (like the flu) rather than psoriasis, for example.

Such an analogy must be used with caution. Traumatic events change people's lives and there may well be an element of managing such changes even though the symptomatology has been reduced successfully. The point is that trauma counselling aims to restore normal functioning, comparable, as nearly as possible, to whatever the person enjoyed prior to the trauma.

Where PTSD has been always a feature of the client's life, such as in the case of early sexual, physical or psychological abuse, such analogies cannot be made and are inappropriate. Client education becomes a matter of not just addressing the experiences and the identities created ('train disaster victim') as there may be no prior 'normal' functioning to restore. In these cases, special attention is needed to the client's future and programmes geared to exploring opportunities and *new* identities for the client to move into that enable him to let go of the past and habituate what to them are normal ways of thinking and feeling. Clients that have never known a 'normal', happy existence should not be deceived into the idea that merely processing past negative experiences alone will automatically create states of being they observe others to enjoy. There are a variety of ways of approaching these additional counselling tasks that are related to TIR models. These are the subject of another book.

In educating the client, overoptimistic expectations should be corrected when found and not reinforced. However, reinforcing the idea that traumas are something that have to be lived with or that symptoms 'can only be managed' is equally non-productive and disempowers clients. We try to give clients realistic hopes and expectations, not false hopes. If a client has no fixed expectations, then the matter does not need to be addressed.

EDUCATING THE CLIENT ON TIR

Counsellors are advised to work out their own ways to explain TIR theory to clients according to the clients' education, experience and their own world views. Metaphors can be very useful as long as they parallel the client's experience. Whatever client education is done, it should result in the following:

- The client understands what you are going to do.
- The client understands what is expected of him.
- The client has no unanswered questions about the counselling activity and the technique you are employing (TIR).

Clients with a knowledge of psychology, counselling or of a sufficient educational level can be given the theory to read from this book or other TIR manuals. Other clients can be given simplified explanations by the counsellor sufficient to meet the above criteria. Described below are some of the concepts we have found to be helpful in educating clients about TIR.

1. A demonstration of the limited attentional capacity (as described in Chapter 2).
2. A demonstration of how much information processing is on automatic and does not require conscious thought, such as driving a familiar route or drinking a cup of tea (as described in Chapter 2). Ask the client how often he has to think about moving a cup of tea to his lips and drinking it without spilling it. Point out that perceptions must be inputted and processed on a sub- or pre-conscious level or he would routinely crash his car or pour tea down his front!

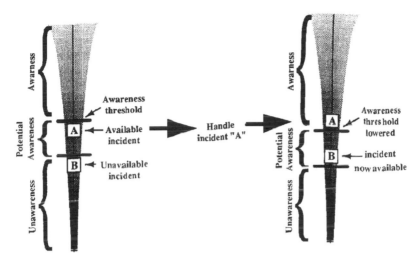

Figure 6: The awareness threshold (Reproduced by kind permission of G. French and F. Gerbode, 1990)

Define pre-conscious memory as information, images, emotions, thoughts which are not currently in consciousness but are accessible to it. Demonstrate the concept by having the client recall the various sights, sounds, smells, emotions, or sensations from an event earlier in the day.

French and Gerbode (1995) use the concept of a threshold of awareness to define pre-conscious and unconscious material (Figure 6). They define the awareness threshold as the dividing line that separates material of which a person can be readily aware (conscious material) from material that is repressed or unconscious. They call the pre-conscious an area of potential awareness and point out that when a pre-conscious issue is brought into awareness and examined, then the awareness threshold lowers. When the threshold lowers, information from the unconscious now moves to the pre-conscious and is therefore available to be examined.

3. Use the analogy of imagining a television programme where the screen is split into many images and all the situations and characters in the story are displayed at once, necessitating replaying it on video many times to make sense of it all.

Use the same analogy to explain TIR: replaying the images like a video machine picking up all the details, the sights, sounds and activities in each frame that attention might not have been paid to at the time of recording or subsequent reflections.

Point out where the video analogy falls down. In a trauma, a person is interactive; even when he is a spectator he is part of the scene and in TIR the counsellor also wants to recover how he felt, what he thought, what he did and didn't do during the incident. (In addition, some clients are not visually oriented so another analogy may need to be chosen or it may be pointed out that it is OK if they don't see images but rather hear the story.)

4. Demonstrate to the client the act of recognition – the fact that he knows what a tea cup is means that it is stored in his memory, which perception of the tea cup triggers. Have the client begin to grasp the concept of cues by having him find an object in the environment that reminds him of an earlier object, incident or activity. Have the client recall a time when he was reminded of earlier incidents by present cues.

5. Explain the idea that traumas can exist in sequences of incidents – earlier incidents being triggered by cues in later incidents. Explain that the 'charge' contained in unprocessed earlier incidents can feed or charge up later ones. Explain that earlier incidents may be either more or less significant than later ones, but that if a sequence exists it is necessary to view the whole of it, latest to earliest. Use the traumatic incident network diagram to explain how incidents can be linked. Point out that the important links might be discerned in counselling but are unlikely to be known about ahead of time, the theory being that if the client really knew the structure of his trauma network, he would be empowered over it rather than suffering from it. No assumptions should be made from the outset as to which incidents might be key-stones in the network.

6. Inform the client that viewing traumatic incidents can be uncomfortable and sometimes quite painful. Emotions and sensations experienced at the time might be re-experienced to a degree. This can be demonstrated by having the client imagine biting into a fresh very sour lemon and asking him to note the sensations in his mouth. Reassure the client that sessions are always taken to a point of completion and that whatever has been triggered in a session has discharged, if not completely, to a point where he is comfortable with it.

7. Explain to the client that information processing may well go on after a session. Bits and pieces might show up, connections might be made or realizations occur. The client should neither deliberately reflect on the session or its content nor prevent himself from automatically doing so. Anything that comes up between sessions will be asked about by the counsellor and acted upon as needed in the next session.

8. Inform the client that trauma counselling is structured to enable him to tackle those incidents that he feels able to examine and process without 're-traumatising' him.

9. Explain the purpose of note-taking and, when needed, get permission to audio tape the sessions and explain the purpose of this. Sometimes this is explained prior to the history-taking. Notes and audio tapes are used for supervisory purposes only.

Issues surrounding confidentiality should be covered prior to the history-taking, in the very beginning of the counselling relationship (usually the first session) as is standard in any counselling setting. We usually cover these issues when we discuss session lengths (as well as fees and payment options if these need to be established).

FITTING THIS METHOD INTO YOUR PRACTICE

One of the most common questions we are asked when we are doing TIR training is how we manage to schedule clients when working with an unfixed session time. Part of how a therapist manages this depends on whether he is working in private practice or in an organization. In private practice, you tend to have more options than when you are working for an organization.

This type of session work can be tiring for both the client and the counsellor; consequently, as counsellors, we do not tend to do more than about six hours of actual session time per day. In our practice, we tend to schedule clients in a variety of ways:

- For the entire day: usually doing two or three sessions
- For the morning: doing either one or two sessions
- For the afternoon: doing either one or two sessions
- For the evening: doing one session
- For intensive work over more than one day.

Sometimes one client is scheduled for intensive work over a few days and another client may be seen for one session in the morning, afternoon or evening when the client doing the intensive work is having a break between sessions. Most clients cannot tolerate more than at most four hours of actual session time in any given day. Unless we are working intensively, most clients will have one session in a day, or possibly two. This is because of the energy required of the client and also because when working with targeted incidents or issues the client may require some time to assimilate and accommodate the information examined in counselling. Although the counsellor may want to cover as much ground as possible, it is VERY important to be sensitive to what an individual can process in any given time. Illuminating information gained from internal sources and brought to consciousness, if not adequately processed within the client's mental capacity, could overwhelm the client. It is equally possible to do too much counselling, past a good end point, as it is to leave issues incomplete (see Chapter 9 for more on this issue).

When working in organizations we tend to schedule clients two hours apart. Clients are made aware that they might have to wait if we run over from our last session, but they are also aware that if they need longer than two hours, we will run over for them. Once the counsellor has done a session or two with the client, she gets an idea of how long the client usually takes to move through material and it is easier to schedule. However, it is unwise to leave less than two hours between TIR sessions, particularly with clients who are dealing with heavy material. The un-fixed session time is one of the most important features of TIR work and it is imperative that clients should not be stopped short of an end point in order to maintain the counsellor's schedule.

Our experience is that ending sessions when an end point has not been reached increases the risk of clients leaving treatment early (e.g., before it is complete). This is particularly true in cases where the counsellor has informed the client that, as often as possible, he will not end the session until an end point has been reached and that session times are unfixed and determined according to process rather than the counsellor's schedule.

In organizations in which other types of counselling are being done by the same therapist, it is wise to schedule TIR sessions for the end of the day so that if the counsellor needs extra time, no clients will be waiting. In our experience, if the organization is made aware of the benefits of TIR and the importance of the longer sessions times, they will be flexible.

Setting fees is another issue that is raised when counsellors first con-sider using this method of working. We recommend that counsellors discuss fees and methods of payment prior to starting any type of coun-selling with the client. When working with unfixed session times or in an intensive manner, this is even more important. Many clients are able to budget for one hour per week for an indefinite period of time (e.g. for a year or two years) to engage in counselling or psychotherapy. It is more difficult for clients to budget for an unknown number of session hours per week (even if the counsellor is only seeing the client once per week) at any fee even if the overall amount of money paid out for counselling is less than what it would have been if it was for one hour per week for two years. For this reason, it is extremely important to be able to offer clients an estimate of final cost and a variety of options for payment of the counsellor's fees.

INTENSIVE WORK VERSUS ONCE WEEKLY WORK

There are advantages and disadvantages to both methods of working. We prefer to see most clients twice per week because there is less time in between sessions for new issues to be triggered by life experience. This makes it possible to resolve some issues piece by piece without having the client become too overwhelmed. If sessions are too far apart, the chances are that many things will arise to trigger new issues in day-to-day life (such as rows with partners, problems at work, and, in many cases with traumatized people, new major traumas such as becoming the victim of another crime).

Some clients can only manage one session in any given day because they need time to integrate their insights between sessions. Other clients can only manage one session per week. For example, clients who have chronic fatigue syndrome often need at least three days to recover from a session because it takes so much mental and physical energy. Frequency of sessions should be tailored to the individual client. Factors for the counsellor to take into account include: convenience factors (distance the client lives from the counsellor's premises, counsellor's schedule, client's schedule), processing style (as mentioned above) and the client's physical condition.

CASE EXAMPLES: MARY AND RENEE

Mary   Mary's work was done intensively — several sessions per day over a weekend. She was seen over three weekends. She wanted to work in this way as she 'want(ed) to get it over with'. She was in good physical health and very motivated to work. In addition, working in this way allowed her to continue her own work as a therapist during the week without any concern that she might be triggered and find it difficult to work. Mary's case was quite complex and we felt that intensive work would allow her to resolve a portion of the trauma network more quickly as life would have less opportunity to provide new triggers. This worked extremely well for Mary and the work took much less time than originally anticipated. In our opinion, had Mary been seen once per week, the total session hours would likely have been double (c.g. 32 instead of 15.5).

Renee   In Renee's case, the trauma was still continuing and there was a considerable amount of upset going on in her life when her counselling began. She was seen twice weekly for most of her work. It would not have been possible to see her more often (e.g. intensively) and probably would not have been useful in the first six weeks of counselling because of all the additional things going on in her life. She needed more time for support in session and to examine the issues going on in the present. If she had been seen once weekly, the work would have taken considerably longer because most of the session time would have been spent dealing with the new triggers and new issues that had arisen in the previous week. Her counselling took about 70 hours and it is speculated that once-weekly sessions would have resulted in at least 150 hours of work.

In our experience, number of traumas does not seem to correspond to number of hours taken in counselling. We have had cases in which there were only two traumas which required 40 hours of work and cases in which there were 40 or more traumas which required 20 hours of work. The length of treatment in part seems to depend on the way in which the client processes information. In addition, it depends on the frequency of sessions, the level of symptomatology, life experiences during the treatment course and individual characteristics of the client. The more experience a counsellor has in working in this way, the easier it becomes to predict how much treatment will be necessary. The average treatment time in cases of Post-Traumatic Stress Disorder (including chronic PTSD) is approximately 20 hours of TIR treatment. Note that this is an average which includes clients such as Mary and Renee who have had multiple traumas.

CREATING A TRAUMA LIST

Following the completion of the history-taking, the counsellor compiles a list of the client's traumas and their dates. The list is then presented to the client for a SUDs (subjective units of distress) rating. A SUDs scale goes from 0 to 10 and the client is asked the following: 'When you think of (incident name here), how distressing is it for you on a scale of 0 to 10 with 0 representing no distress at all and 10 being the maximum distress?' The client is told that this is not an exact science but simply a way of gaining some idea of how, at present, these traumas might impact on him.

Clients sometimes experience some confusion in SUDs ratings between the impact of the incident at the time and how they feel about it in the present. The counsellor can have the client make two ratings: (1) the impact at the time of the incident – how distressing it was then; (2) how distressing it is now.

In our experience, the presenting trauma that prompted the client to request counselling turns out not to be the one that has greatest impact. It is very often the case that the latest incident in a trauma network (and the initial presenting issue), although in itself quite substantial, is primarily a trigger for earlier incidents. It is the one that, together with a preceding sequence of traumatic events, the client's mental defences were not able to cope with and overwhelmed them. This is not always the case, but in practice it makes no difference to procedure. Having obtained the SUDs rating, the counsellor informs the client that it is entirely up to him which incident is addressed first. The client may choose (and usually does) an incident with a low SUDs rating. Whatever the client chooses, the counsellor will address and proceed through the list in the same way until trauma counselling is complete.

SUDs ratings allow a client to assess and exercise choice in what is addressed and in what order. As a rule of thumb, it enables the counsellor to know that the client's interest in a particular trauma means that it has significance and substance for the client and benefit will be gained from addressing it. It also usually means that it will be within the client's capacity to confront and to talk about its content without being too distressed or completely overwhelmed by it.

However, in our experience, SUDs ratings are often an inaccurate way of determining the severity of charge encapsulated in a trauma. Despite thorough assessments, clients (and counsellors) are often surprised that what was initially thought to be a SUDs rating of '2' turns out to be '9' when it is addressed. An explanation for this is that the negative contents of an individual's mental environment have been subject to defences, and notwithstanding their failure (resulting in trauma symptomatology), they remain to some extent in place. Given that the charge encysted in these incidents has been suppressed or repressed, the extent of it is unknown to the client (and counsellor). Moreover, it is the client's unawareness of how his trauma network is connected and which of his experiences are keystones in the network that necessitates counselling in the first place. In a nutshell, if the client knew what was wrong with him, it wouldn't be wrong with him or he would already be dealing with it.

As individual traumas are addressed, a counsellor can expect the initial SUDs ratings to change. Incidents the client thought were heavily charged and significant may now become less significant and other incidents previously written off as having little or no impact are realized to be of major consequence. SUDs ratings seem to be highly subject to change and, rather than an accurate indicator of the substance of a trauma, should be regarded as a device to enable the client to reflect on and choose which part of her own material should next be addressed.

As each trauma is addressed to an end point, it is ticked off as such, together with those addressed because they were part of a sequence. When the entire list has been addressed, it can be represented to the client for another SUDs rating. This would only be done if the counsellor or client has doubts about how effective the counselling has been to date. In this case, the client is invited to reflect again on each trauma and rate it. Additional counselling procedures would then be planned in the event that the client feels that some of the traumas still impact on them (see Chapter 7, thematic TIR).

If SUDs ratings are used at all (and they can be omitted altogether), at no time should they be used to determine whether an end point or point of resolution has been reached, or in any manner that might give the client the idea that she is expected to reduce them.

Examples of Trauma Lists from Mary and Renee

Mary

Incident name	SUDs	Addressed?
Father in caravan	10	Yes
Mother beating sister	8	Yes
Assault by client	5	Yes
Sexual assault by doctor	10	Yes
Date rape attempted	10	No interest
Second sexual assault by doctor	10	Yes
Father tried to kill me	10	Yes
Kitchen table incident	10	Yes
Beatings by mother	6	No interest
Confronting father about abuse	5	No interest
Sexual abuse by father	10	Yes
Mother leaving father	8	Yes
Incident with sister over relationship with father	5	No interest
Possible ectopic pregnancy	10	No interest
Father raped mother	5	Yes
Grandmother's death	10	Yes
Teacher beat girl	3	No interest
Attempted molest by priest	4	No interest
Friend killed in accident	5	Yes
Operation incident	7	Yes
Throat operation	9	Yes
Gas mask incident	9	Yes
Witness car accident	4	No interest
Father in fight	3	Yes
Incident on table	10	Yes
Bombing incident	2	Yes

Renee

Date of trauma	Incident name	SUDs	Addressed?
1953	Nan and aunt fought in passage	2	No interest
1957	Loss of mother	6	Yes
1965	Prevented from getting job	1	Yes
1964	Dad spending savings	4	Yes
1966	Son adopted	8	Yes
1981	Death of Roger's father	5	Yes
1983	Angela starts taking drugs	10	Yes
1987	George starts taking drugs	10	Yes
1989	Death of mother-in-law	7	Yes
1991	Death of father	10	No interest
1993	Threatened with shotgun	10	Yes
1994	Car accident	9	Yes
1982	Suicide attempt	10	Yes
1995	Kicked out George	10	No interest
1970	Burgled	3	Yes
1979	Mugged	3	Yes
1985	Assaulted by Roger	10	Yes
1966	Used by boyfriend	5	Yes
1964	Prevented from going to drama school	3	Yes
1989	Loss of friend	2	Yes
1982	Death of cousin	6	Yes
1995	Shot by Roger	10	Yes
1957–59	Period staying with nan and aunt	10	No interest
1959 65	Period staying with dad and stepmother	10	No interest

Note: For those marked 'No interest' – towards the end of counselling, the client was asked to go over the list and stated no interest in looking at these incidents.

In the following chapter, we examine what the counsellor does at the beginning of each session, and look in more depth at the process of using the trauma list to pick the first item that will be worked on with TIR or Unblocking.

5

CHOOSING WHICH INCIDENT TO WORK ON FIRST

In the previous chapter, we covered the steps that are necessary before beginning the actual TIR and related techniques which is the body of the therapeutic work. These steps are integral to the counselling process as they establish the rules and context of the trauma work. Having provided a context, in this chapter we examine the procedure at the beginning of the session, the format of keeping notes for a session, and how to choose which incident is addressed first. If we compare the course of counselling to a story having a beginning, a middle and an end, the previous chapter covered the beginning of the counselling story, and this chapter begins its middle.

THE BEGINNING OF THE SESSION

Sessions usually begin by asking about, and addressing as needed, three areas:

A. The client's physical ability to engage in the session. This should include amount and quality of sleep the previous night, whether or not the client has eaten recently, and any drugs or alcohol consumed in the past 24 hours.

B. The client's present circumstances and concerns.

C. Anything that has occurred since the last session that the client's attention might be on. This includes any upsets, problems, information the client wants to communicate, questions and insights.

Counsellors are advised to use whatever questions they are comfortable with to explore these areas. Examples for A might include: 'How are you today?', 'How much sleep did you get last night?', 'Are you hungry at the moment?', 'Have you had any drugs or alcohol in the past 24 hours?'. Examples for B might include: 'Is anything bothering you right now?', 'Is there anything your attention is presently caught up on?'. Examples for C might include: 'How have you been doing since I last saw you?', 'Has anything upsetting happened?', 'Is there anything that has been worrying you?', 'Has anything occurred that you feel you should tell me about?', 'Did you have any thoughts about our last session?', 'Did you have any questions you wanted to ask me?'.

The idea is to explore, as needed anything the client's attention is on, get up to date on any relevant developments in the client's life and ensure that the client is able and ready to continue the counselling programme. Sometimes it is necessary to amend the programme based on what the client presents at the beginning of the session. The emphasis here is on clearing up anything the client's attention is *already on* and not to trigger issues that are not live or current. Over-exploring the initial questions can result in triggering issues that were not live before, therefore extending the client's counselling. Under-exploring the initial questions can result in continuing a counselling programme when a client is preoccupied with current or recent issues or events (which seldom works because the client's attention is on those events, not on the issue he is addressing in the session).

Particularly when clients are receiving regular and frequent sessions, they may only need relatively brief or cursory enquiries to establish that they are ready to continue their counselling programme where they left off. In some cases, life events may mean that an entire session is spent dealing with a particular issue the client is absorbed with in the present. In this case there is no option but to suspend the planned programme until another time.

'Exploring' issues which show up during the initial questions means discussing them with the client to a place of comfort – a point at which the client's attention is now off that subject, or if actions are necessary to deal with an issue then decisions are made on how and when these actions will be taken.

Decisions about the client's physical ability to engage in a session must be made carefully. If a client is overtired, hungry or has used alcohol or drugs within 24 hours of the session, he is unlikely to have the mental and physical energy to engage in a TIR session to a good point of resolution. (One glass of wine – i.e. 1 unit of alcohol – or one aspirin will not interfere in the session. However, abstaining entirely is always best.) Considerable concentration and focus are needed on the part of the client to engage in a TIR session, and this requires energy. (These issues were discussed in depth in Chapter 3.) The counsellor needs to get enough information at the beginning of the session to make a decision as to whether to proceed with TIR and related techniques, to focus on present issues, or to suspend the session altogether.

GUIDE TO NOTE-TAKING IN TIR AND RELATED SESSIONS

Notes are taken simultaneously with counselling rather than written up afterwards. Clients with previous experience of counselling where this wasn't done may find it a little different and have to adjust to this difference in style. On the other hand, our experience is that most clients appreciate that what they say is being noted as well as heard. They should be informed in their education that the reason for extensive notes is to ensure that their counselling programme can be tailored to suit them and that issues are neither forgotten nor addressed twice in error (as well as for supervisory purposes).

History notes are most important as treatment planning is conducted from these. The form should be completed with this in mind, therefore clear, legible handwriting is essential. In TIR sessions, the emphasis is on noting what was addressed, how it was addressed and how it went. Notes should contain the client's name and the date, any issues brought up and addressed at the beginning of the session, the incident(s) addressed including when and where they occurred (this includes any earlier incidents), use of any additional questions, any issues that came up that may need to be addressed in a later session, and any questions or comments the client has at the end of the session. If a theme was addressed then it should be noted exactly as the client worded it. The same is true for an Unblocking subject.

Whatever system of note-taking counsellors use, it should be adequate to provide a picture of the client's counselling and facilitate the counsellor's supervision. Initially, when counsellors are first learning to use TIR and related techniques, it is useful if they note what they say in session as well as what the client says in session. This makes it easier for the supervisor to see the pattern of the session and often makes it possible for the supervisor to pinpoint errors.

CHOOSING INCIDENTS TO ADDRESS

After educating the client in TIR procedure in detail, as described in the previous chapter, TIR can begin provided that sufficient session time is available. When you use TIR with a client for the first time, do not begin the procedure on an incident if there is less than 90 minutes session time available. The counsellor does not decide what incident the client will address. The SUDs rated trauma list is placed before the client and he is informed that he may pick out any incident to address regardless of how it has been SUDs rated. A typical question might be: 'Which of these incidents are you most interested in addressing first? It doesn't matter whether you choose one that you have rated as heavily charged or one that seemed to be lightly charged.' Another option is: 'Do any of these incidents jump off the page as urgently needing attention? It doesn't matter how they were rated when we did the SUDs.' Take the incident that *the client wants* to address and use TIR to address it.

We earlier described that the client is unlikely to have a correct idea of how significant individual incidents are in affecting his life and his trauma network. Although we still recommend the use of SUDs ratings to enable the client to get an idea of how heavy and significant he may think an incident is, experience has shown that the client is often wrong. For example, one client chose an incident that she rated as a 2 (when there were many 8, 9 and 10 ratings on her list) as a light incident to start off with. This incident when addressed proved to be one of the most heavily charged on her list. Though exceptional, this happens often enough to be worthy of mention. Conversely, an incident thought to be heavily charged can turn out to be much lighter than initially expected. For example, Mary chose an incident that she rated a 9 and when she addressed it, it turned out to be quite lightly charged.

In general, the client's interest and choice of incidents guarantees their ability to confront and process it. Clients usually can be relied upon to pick incidents that will not overwhelm them in session. Therefore, it is crucial that counsellors create a safe space in which clients can not only address their traumas but retain the power of choice over what they choose to examine.

When the first incident has been addressed successfully and an end point reached, then the procedure is repeated afresh each session. The trauma list is again placed before the client and the next incident is chosen, and so on.

Occasionally, a client might start with a lightly charged incident which proves to be connected to a sequence of earlier incidents (which may or may not be on the list) that are much more heavily charged. In this instance there is little choice but to address them with TIR. To date, this has never been found to be a problem – the clients have always come through, but in the event that any clients feel unable to examine an earlier incident the counsellor should never coerce them. Other, lighter incidents can be addressed first or a gradient approach can be used (see Chapter 7).

In our experience, it has never been necessary to address every incident on the trauma list. Some will be found to be of no interest and will not need addressing at all. Quite often the client, having addressed a majority of incidents, reaches an end point for the trauma counselling. This is often characterized as no longer having PTSD symptoms and the client's attention is now on the present and future rather than on the past. Such shifts are unmistakable when they occur and trauma counselling can be ended at that time. We schedule at least one follow-up session to ensure the stability of the results.

If the client has experienced previous counselling, it might be necessary to explore this or unblock that counselling. This is particularly important when the client has had negative experiences in counselling so that the client can put those experiences in the past and doesn't carry negative expectations forward into the present counselling relationship. We suggest this as a place to start when clients have had previous counselling, but if they have no interest in this activity we then move on to the main body of the work.

Because of Mary's considerable previous experience of counselling, the counsellor started with an Unblocking on previous counselling. Mary was very interested in doing this and the session went extremely well. She reached an end point for that session which included a strong feeling that this new counselling relationship was different from the ones that she had previously experienced and that any negative experiences she had had were now in the past. She said 'It's like having a clean slate'.

Unblocking addresses positive and negative elements of a subject or experience. It is essential that benefits from previous counselling are not invalidated. Unblocking (and educating the client about unblocking) is dealt with in depth in the next chapter.

6

USING UNBLOCKING

As described in Chapter 1, Unblocking is a counselling procedure that uses repetition to produce a reduction of emotional charge and cognitive clarification for a specific area of difficulty. The counsellor can use Unblocking successfully with an area in the client's life where TIR would be less effective or inappropriate. It is often used to get the client ready for TIR – helping the client to defuse situations that exist for him in his present life. In TIR, especially basic TIR, the counsellor asks the client to focus on past, heavily charged events. If his attention is on a relationship or problem of immediate concern (usually something that is ongoing), he will not be able to focus on these past events until the immediate problem is addressed. For example, if the client is in danger of losing his job, he is unlikely to be able to focus on a past traumatic event until his safety has been addressed. The same is true if a client is having extreme problems in his marital relationship. He may be unable to examine previous traumas until he feels reasonably secure that he will still have a marital relationship when he returns home that night.

A counsellor can use Unblocking to address relationships with specific people or specific situations on which her client's attention is fixed. Examples of Unblocking topics include: relationship with wife, husband, sister, mother, difficulties at work, travelling to work, writing a book and meeting a deadline. Any topic that is not a discreet traumatic incident can be examined in this fashion (in conjunction with any other intervention that may be needed).

Unblocking is a counselling procedure designed to enable a client to examine a specific issue he has by taking it apart piecemeal, using a list of questions that are asked repeatedly. The idea is one of unpeeling the layers of the issue, therefore being able to examine it in some depth from different viewpoints.

If a person is faced with a stressful situation – e.g. incoming information of a quantity or quality that cannot be processed consciously or successfully, then mental defence mechanisms are automatically used to cope with it. Most of us are familiar with the Freudian concept of 'repression' – the automatic 'parking' of some uncomfortable emotion, idea or perception. Unblocking consists of a list of questions calculated to uncover how a person has construed and 'dealt with' a problematic issue in her life and mental environment whether consciously accomplished or by means of unconscious, automatic defence mechanisms.

When a client's methods of assimilating and accommodating a situation, event or problem are successful at dealing with it – regardless of how this is accomplished – then there should be no negative implications for his mental health. That such an issue remains live, absorbing his attention or is 'charged', illustrates that whatever methods (or defences) were employed have failed to deal with the issue. Unblocking consists of systematically examining how the issue was 'dealt with' in order to facilitate insight into it, reconstruing it and discharging its negative effects.

Many forms of counselling involve the counsellor evaluating how the client has tried to make sense of her issues and used her mental defences, necessitating the counsellor thinking and posing questions calculated to expose and address what the client has actually been doing with the issue. By having a list of questions to use and refer to, a counsellor does not have to rely on his intuition, experience, and skill in the session to formulate questions, but rather can place more of his attention on the client. Furthermore, regardless of how skilled the counsellor, he, like the client, will have his own blindspots. The use of a list of questions enables the counsellor to cover possible constructions that he and his client may not think of during a session. Thus, the use of these questions can broaden an analysis of any of the client's issues and ease the 'brain strain' of the counsellor.

The lists of unblocking questions have evolved over several years of experience. They are thought to include most of the usual things a person might do with a problematical issue. Obviously, some of these questions might not make sense to individual clients and the questions may need to be reworded for particular clients. Counsellors may think of other possible questions which could be added. When this is done, the counsellors are advised to ensure that any additional questions are as non-suggestive as possible. Client education on unblocking includes informing him that these are generic questions, some of which may be relevant to his issue and some not so. These are questions, not statements, calculated to enable him to discharge any negative effects of the issue and help *him* analyse it.

Unblocking can be used to address almost any intimate or environmental concern the client might have that is preventing him from focusing on TIR, or it can be used on its own to address these types of concerns. In the case of environmental problems, Unblocking can be used to defuse the issue prior to helping the client to formulate an action plan. For example: The client feels he is not getting appropriate medical attention and is upset, worried, confused and feels powerless about it. One approach might be to Unblock 'Regarding your medical treatment . . . '. Once this was completed and the area was discharged, then together the counsellor and client could figure out what the client actually needs to do to remedy any actual situation in the world that requires attention (e.g. speak to his GP, change his GP, seek a second opinion, etc.).

Our experience has been that Unblocking results in a variety of types of resolution or end points:

1. The client feels the issue has been completely resolved and has no further attention on it. (This type of end point should be achievable when Unblocking has been used to address a recent upset, for example.)
2. The client feels much better about the issue and knows how to deal with it now and so his attention is not now on it. (This type of end point is typical of when the issue has an environmental component and action is needed.)
3. The client feels better, has not resolved the issue but now has it much more clearly defined, enabling the counsellor and client to plan and implement further interventions to address the issue. (This type of end point is typical of when the issue is a core issue, complex issue or a long-standing issue.)

Almost any of the client's issues can be addressed with Unblocking, with the provision that *specific* issues are addressed that avoid the danger of dismantling all of the client's defence mechanisms and overwhelming her. For example, you might unblock your 'relationship with Mary' but you would not unblock 'your problems in life' as that would obviously trigger many issues at once and not resolve any of them. With clients that the counsellor knows well and who have good ego strength, more general issues can be safely addressed such as 'Regarding work' or 'Concerning your sexuality'.

UNBLOCKING PROCEDURE

The Unblocking lists consist of concepts: each concept is a way in which the client might have dealt with the issue (either consciously or unconsciously). For example: if a person becomes angry with her partner when in public, she might suppress the anger rather than express it because of concerns about 'making a scene'.

There are two lists of Unblocking concepts and sample questions. Counsellors should choose the one that is most appropriate in length, depending on how substantial the client's issue appears to be. For example, if a client's recent upset is being addressed the shorter list should be adequate. If the issue is more substantial or long standing, such as an intimate relationship, then the longer list would be chosen. In any event, if some point of resolution is not obtained with the shorter list then the longer one can be used. The shorter list of concepts with sample questions is included in this chapter. The longer list can be found in Appendix 2. Unblocking steps are applied using the framework discussed in Chapter 1 with the rules for this method, including the specific communication style. The procedure is as follows:

1. Begin with the client's issue, making sure that it is an issue that he is interested in addressing. For example, at the beginning of the session the client tells the counsellor that she is extremely upset about her relationship with her mother and 'cannot think of anything else'.

2. Check the wording of the issue and use whatever brief wording that the *client* feels encapsulates the issue. For example: the client has been describing a problem with his girlfriend in that he resents her going to clubs with her friends without him. The counsellor would explore the area with the client to establish what he would call that problem. It might be 'jealousy', 'a feeling of rejection', 'my girlfriend's behaviour' or something else. Try to get a succinct item but *use the client's wording of it*.

3. Having obtained the wording, use the appropriate unblocking list to address it. Take the first concept and formulate a question to *fit the item*. For example, 'What effect has this feeling of rejection had on you?' or 'How has jealousy impacted on you?'. The concepts are there for the counsellor to incorporate into his own preferred language, taking into account what the client will understand easily, his language, and his culture. The list later in this chapter is written in question form as an example. It is not important how the question is phrased, as long as it can be understood by the client and the **counsellor does not vary the wording each time he asks the question.**

4. 'Soak' the question or concept by repeating it until the client has no more answers to it, being sure to acknowledge answers already given. For example: 'OK. Are there any other effects this jealousy has had on you?' If the counsellor is not clear about what the client is expressing, then he can reiterate what the client has said so far and check that he understands. Otherwise, use of reflection is not helpful as it interrupts the flow of the procedure (e.g. the client must keep moving his attention from his own material to the counsellor and back to his own material). The same is true when the counsellor varies the wording of the question each time. This interrupts the flow of the session and is not advised.

Remember that the issue being addressed is one that has been a source of confusion or distress to the client and he is consulting the counsellor for the purpose of arriving at some sort of certainty from the midst of uncertainty and confusion. The imposition of a structure and completing each component part of it facilitates that process. By repeatedly examining a concept from different angles, the client is enabled to see what specific relevance that concept has compared to the relevance it does not have. For example:

COUNSELLOR: How has jealousy affected you?
CLIENT: It has made me miserable whenever my girlfriend went out with her friends. I felt terrible. I couldn't stop imagining what she might be up to.
COUNSELLOR: OK. How has jealousy affected you?
CLIENT: It has made me question everything she does. I've been uptight and not able to relax until I'm satisfied that she didn't do anything I would be jealous of.
COUNSELLOR: OK. Is there any other way jealousy has affected you?
CLIENT (*after some thought*): No that's it. (*insight*) It's in those specific instances, it not something I generally have a problem with. It is only when she is out with her friends.

Here the point is that the client has not been left in a state of uncertainty by being asked about a negative condition without it being explored to the point of being able to identify its parameters before moving on. The idea in Unblocking is that (ideally – and it will not be evident in every question) a concept is explored to some point of conclusion before going on to another question. Experienced counsellors may think this is self-evident but the rationale deserves a mention. It is so easy to ask about various elements of a client's experience without the provision of at least defusing issues if not concluding with insight.

5. Having soaked a question to a conclusion, go on to the next question and continue until an end point has been reached on the subject. From a process point of view this might consist of: (1) no further answers to questions are forthcoming; (2) the client has experienced an insight into the problem that appears conclusive (at least for now); (3) the client has become bored with the subject by virtue of having discharged it and is no longer interested in it.

Usually, the exploration of a significant and substantial issue with Unblocking results in an unmistakable end point: a reconstruction of the issue following an insight or cognitive shift. At this point the Unblocking is ended whether only one or two questions or the whole of a list has been used. The other evidence of an end point is also often present: the client's attention turns from his mental environment to the external environment and the client is looking and feeling better. If no end point is reached then a further list can be used or the same list can be worked over again. (Awareness changes from doing it once, and can mean that further information may be available on the second time through.) Obviously, if the client answers 'No' or 'Nothing comes to mind' to a question, you move on to the next question.

BASIC LIST OF CONCEPTS – INCLUDING SAMPLE QUESTIONS

What follows is the basic list of concepts used for Unblocking (along with some synonyms). The concepts are in **bold** type embedded in the questions. The counsellor should construct appropriate questions using words that the client is likely to understand. Synonyms are in brackets. The counsellor should choose one word to represent the concept and keep that constant each time the question is asked. For example, if the counsellor had chosen to use 'helpless' instead of 'powerless' for the second question, then each time he asked the question he should have used 'helpless'.

Make sure to phrase questions so that they suit the subject the client chooses to address and are not awkward. Make sure to mention the issue chosen each time the question is asked, as this helps to keep the client on track. For example, 'Regarding your relationship with your sister, have you suppressed anything?', 'Regarding your relationship with your sister, have you suppressed anything else?', 'Regarding your relationship with your sister, have you felt powerless?'.Where (subject) appears in the questions below, it refers to the issue the client has chosen.

0. How has (subject) **affected** you?
   Include effects on client's feelings, attitudes, activities, view of self, relationship with others.

1. Regarding (subject), have you **suppressed** anything? (buried, bottled up, 'parked')
2. Regarding (subject), have you felt **powerless**? (helpless)
3. Regarding (subject), have you **distanced** yourself from anything or anyone? (separated from, withdrawn from, avoided)
4. Regarding (subject), have you been **worried** about something? (concerned about, anxious about, troubled you)

5. Regarding (subject), have you been **wary** of anything or anyone? (cautious about, careful about)
6. Regarding (subject), has anything been **misunderstood**? (misconstrued, misinterpreted)
7. Regarding (subject), has anything been **disregarded**? (ignored, sidelined)
8. Regarding (subject), has a **judgement** been made? (evaluated, assessed, put a value on)
9. Regarding (subject), has anything been **concealed**? (hidden, withheld)
10. Regarding (subject), has anything been **denied**? (failed to admit, failed to confront)
11. Regarding (subject), has anything been **disagreed** with? (objected to, protested)
12. Regarding (subject), has anything been **proposed**? (suggested, advised, instructed)
13. Regarding (subject), has anything been **incomprehensible**? (illogical, unfathomable, nonsensical)
14. Regarding (subject), has there been a **failure**? (loss, disappointment)
15. Regarding (subject), has anything not been **acknowledged**? (not given credit for, minimized)
16. Regarding (subject), has anything been **negated**? (dismissed, thought unimportant)
17. Regarding (subject), is there anything you **felt strongly about**? (asserted, stated strongly)
18. Regarding (subject), has a **mistake** been made? (misjudgement, incorrect solution)
19. Regarding (subject), has there been a **dilemma**? (problem, conflict)
20. Regarding (subject), was anything **forced on** you? (compelled you to do or accept)
21. Regarding (subject), has anyone been **blamed** for something? (accused, held responsible for)
22. Regarding (subject), has there been a **compromise**? (concession, bargain)
23. Regarding (subject), has anything been **desired**? (wanted, coveted)
24. Regarding (subject), has anything been **concluded**? (deduced, inferred, assumed)
25. Regarding (subject), have you **restrained** yourself from doing or saying anything? (held back)
26. Regarding (subject), are you **missing information**?
27. Regarding (subject), has some **responsibility** not been admitted? (fault, obligation, duty)
28. Regarding (subject), is there something you have not been able to **control**? (master)

29. Regarding (subject), is there an aspect of it that has been **advantageous**? (beneficial, profitable)
30. Regarding (subject), is there something you have **not acted** upon? (have not done)
31. Regarding (subject), has anything been **revealed**? (exposed, unveiled)
32. Regarding (subject), have any **decisions** been made? (conclusions, resolutions)
33. Regarding (subject), is there anything that ought to be **changed**? (altered, modified, transformed)
34. Regarding (subject), is there anything that has been **overlooked**? (neglected, disregarded)
35. Regarding (subject), has anything been **achieved**? (accomplished, attained)

If Unblocking does not work well, then it may be for the following reasons:

1. The issue or item was not of sufficient interest or importance to the client in the first place.
2. The counsellor's language in using the concepts was not understandable to the client.
3. Unblocking was not an appropriate procedure, i.e. the client either expected or needed some other approach.

Unblocking has been widely used for some years and found to be broadly useful. In the event that a counsellor finds it doesn't suit a client and 'goes nowhere' then the above factors can be explored with the client and some other approach utilized.

Occasionally, Unblocking uncovers something that requires a different approach. For example, while unblocking jealousy the client remembers a very painful early incident of rejection by a girlfriend that really requires TIR. In this instance, the counsellor would switch to TIR, complete that and then return to Unblocking. (Usually, Unblocking is returned to in the next session as an end point is reached on the TIR). Another possibility: While unblocking jealousy the client realizes that he has possibly completely misconstrued something his girlfriend said and needs to talk to her. In this instance the counsellor might decide to end the session to enable the client to discuss it with her. He would then return to the subject in a later session to complete the unblocking as necessary.

In some situations, a subject area is of such significance and complexity that an unblocking of the whole area may take several sessions. In these instances, an end point is often reached for each session and then new material examined in the subsequent sessions until the client feels the area is resolved.

It is expected that counsellors will devise their own questions around the concepts in deference to their client's educational level, language and cultural background and that they will add any additional questions that they think may be appropriate. Counsellors should beware of adding questions, emphasizing existing ones or putting them in a way that leads a client. No one question should be asked any differently from any another.

With Unblocking, as with TIR, it is important that the client brings up whatever comes to his mind when the question is asked. The questions act as keystones – a place to start deconstructing old concepts and constructing new more appropriate ones. Sometimes the client's answers do not seem to fit the questions – but as long as there is change and movement (e.g. processing is occurring) then this does not matter. As with TIR and other related techniques, the counsellor must be process-oriented rather than content-oriented. The content of what the client is saying is important in as much as it lets the counsellor know where in the process the client is at a given moment, and gives the counsellor clues as to what he should do next (e.g. move to the next concept, ask the same question, ask for clarification or end the session). The counsellor should beware of attaching significance to a particular insight or interpretation made by the client. For example, a counsellor may believe that forgiveness is an important step in a client recovering from abuse. He should not be looking for the client to come up with a statement or insight that indicates that she forgives the person who abused her in order to decide when the end point has been reached. Some clients may well forgive their abusers and others may not. As long as the cognitive shift is accompanied by the other signs of an end point (indicating it is an adaptive one for the client at that time) then the counsellor should end the Unblocking procedure. Remember, the object of Unblocking is to facilitate the client's process of deconstructing an area and then reconstructing it. This is a process and the content will be different for each client.

AN EXAMPLE OF UNBLOCKING

Here we present an example of Unblocking. In this session, Jane's attention is on a relationship she had with Eric some years before. This was the first Unblocking session that Jane had during her counselling. Prior to this, she had completed 12 sessions of TIR. The counsellor's questions are in regular print and Jane's responses are in *italics*. The counsellor's observations are also in regular print in brackets. Note that the concepts and their order have been revised since this session was done, so the concepts used in this excerpt differ from the sample list earlier in the chapter. In any event, the counsellor would word the concept using whatever synonym the client is most comfortable with.

Jane's Unblocking Session: In Terms of Her Relationship with Eric

In terms of your relationship with Eric, have you suppressed anything?

Not deliberately in the present. At the time, I didn't talk to anyone about the relationship. Now, I'm talking with you about it and I have talked about it to friends.

OK. In terms of your relationship with Eric, have you suppressed anything?

No. That's fine.

Fine. In terms of your relationship with Eric, has anything or anyone been belittled?

Don't know. Yes. The friendship between us. The truth. In real terms as to what happened. It's like in a book – reading a script taken out of context. We had faith and belief. Eric took them to use for control and power – as faith can be used – to extend one individual's power. It's not a living truth. When I was seeing Dr Flowers – Eric's behaviour belittled my growth.

OK. In terms of your relationship with Eric, has anything else been belittled?

I belittled my own self – thinking that perhaps Eric was right in terms of what he was saying – the things he quoted. I belittled myself and my own faith and this has invalidated me as a human being. (Jane is speaking in an angry tone. Body posture is rigid.) *Yes. I belittled myself as a human being who had the right to live as an independent person. The gift I had been given through my work with Dr Flower – going to university – a gift for people – not something one person could own, control, contained. Whenever I did get a job, within three days he would show up – drunk, extremely wrecked – pathetic. I lost the job. I was so angry – anything I did he destroyed. Ultimately – he would destroy my life. I belittled my healthy angry feelings.*

Got it. In terms of your relationship with Eric, has anything else been belittled?

Yes. When I tried to tell people that I was attacked and in danger. They heard me but didn't hear me. The scale didn't register. It was not particularly their fault.

I hadn't realized how difficult it is for people to hear something horrendous has happened. Only a few people can hear you. It affected trying to get some help – when the helpers didn't hear I felt worthless – It affected every area of my life. When they asked me to leave the group it put me in danger of being killed by Eric. I wouldn't go to any events where I felt he might be there.

OK. In terms of your relationship with Eric, has anything else been belittled?

All things – as an emerging woman – not just by him but through others as well. Things to do with my culture, my intelligence. Everything. No area that wasn't. The awful thing is I went along with some of it. (Jane is speaking in a calm tone, looking more relaxed in body posture). *That's all.*

OK. In terms of your relationship with Eric, has anything or anyone been judged?

Yes. Morally, spiritually, the lot. My behaviour, my choices. By other people, by myself – against God's standards of commandments but without grace. Judged and found wanting. (Jane had tears running down her face.)

OK. In terms of your relationship with Eric, has anything else or anyone else been judged?

Yes. I've judged his behaviour and his effect on me and wanted him dead. To come by some justice. But not want him to come before people as judge but rather go before God as judge. People would tear him to shreds. God judges with mercy. I judged myself and although I wasn't judged by my family – I felt I was. (Jane is no longer crying. Her body posture is relaxed.)

OK. In terms of your relationship with Eric, have any other judgements been made?

Nothing else.

Fine. In terms of your relationship with Eric, is there anything you've been wary about?

(Jane laughs.) *That my birth control was taken care of. What I said to people, what I wanted, who I told anything about it. I thought no one can love someone who has been so horrendous. Not talking to anyone who might talk to Eric. Well-meaning people would let him know where I was, what I was doing – all in the name of love and not realize they were putting me in danger.* (Jane laughs.) *I was extremely cynical – to protect myself. To look after myself. It would have been healthier to shoot him.* (Jane laughs.) *I couldn't have though. Nothing else.*

OK. In terms of your relationship with Eric, has anything been concealed?

I'd like to know if he'd ever done the things he said he'd done. It was most of him. I feel as if I've been revealed in everything – exposed things still secret. When you are so open a funny thing happens – you can see where everyone else is. (Jane laughs. Body posture quite relaxed. Normal facial colour.) *I come from a different place now. That's all.*

Fine. In terms of your relationship with Eric, is there anything that has been resisted?

Communication – all of it. Taking care of the boundaries. This was something he couldn't understand. He wanted to have a battle. I simply wanted to relax. Nobody could put the pieces together. I made the choice to come here for help. So I didn't have to live with it anymore – not be overwhelmed. Feel like I could handle it – can make choices and positive choices. I feel certain of this – the relationship is over and now I can let go of it. I can protect myself and can make better choices because I'm not holding onto it. (Jane speaking in a relaxed tone, relaxed body posture, smiling.)

OK. How does this feel at the moment?

Good. Finished. Like I've cleared the stuff away and have made new decisions. Whole.

Is there anything you would like to add before we end?

No. That's fine.

(End of excerpt.)

Note that the counsellor ended the session after the sixth concept had been explored, when there was ample evidence of an end point having been reached. In this case, Jane was smiling, laughing, making eye contact with the counsellor, and speaking about the relationship as being finished, speaking about the future and reporting feeling whole. When she began the session, the relationship felt unfinished, in the present, and still influencing her life and her decisions. Not all Unblocking sessions go this well but when they don't resolve issues, they nearly always clarify them.

In general, Unblocking is versatile and easy to use. It provides a client with a structure that enables them to access, explore and process their issues and provides counsellors with a procedure by which they do not have to rely solely on their intuition or cognitive processes in session to address a client's issues.

CORRECTING UNBLOCKING IN THE SAME SESSION

Some of the reasons for Unblocking sessions not going well were covered earlier in this chapter. The most common errors in Unblocking are covered here.

Not Spending Long Enough on Each Concept

The counsellor should move on to the next concept if:

1. The client says there are no more answers to a particular concept.
2. There is a cognitive shift and new insight on a concept is achieved.
3. There is no further change on a concept (e.g. the client says 'that is all').

If the answers to a concept are changing, the counsellor should continue examining the same concept.

Missing the End Point

Because end points in Unblocking can sometimes be more subtle (e.g. the client just loses interest in the subject), counsellors can more easily miss the end point. If the Unblocking is on a recent upset, then the counsellor should not expect a major insight or cognitive shift on the area. If the counsellor misses the end point, he should follow the procedure detailed under the section on missing the end point in TIR in Chapter 9.

Forgetting to Return to Unblocking after Completing a TIR Item that Arose During an Unblocking

If an incident arises during Unblocking that needs to be examined with TIR, the counsellor shifts to TIR until the incident is resolved. The counsellor must then remember to check with the client in the next session to see if the area being examined in Unblocking has been completed. If it has not, the counsellor resumes the unblocking where he left off in the last session. It is the counsellor's job to make sure that any area he starts examining with the client is completed. Part of maintaining the client's safety is ensuring that compartmented areas are addressed to a point of completion before moving on to other areas.

The Client was Distracted by Something Else

This is the same as with TIR and is detailed in Chapter 9.

The Client is Withholding Something from the Counsellor

Again, this is the same as with TIR and is detailed in Chapter 9. Long pauses before the client answers 'No' to a question sometimes indicate that the client is thinking about, but not voicing, material and it is worth checking with the client before moving on to the next concept.

7

WORKING WITH
TRAUMATIC INCIDENTS

TIR has a number of different applications. In this book, we cover the two most commonly used: basic TIR and thematic TIR. In previous chapters, we presented the theory behind TIR. In this chapter, we cover the practical theory and the actual TIR counselling steps. These steps are applied in the framework discussed earlier in the book – using the rules for this method including the communication style, which were all described in Chapter 1.

BASIC TIR

Basic TIR methodology is used when a client has identified and presented a specific traumatic incident (or a group of specific incidents). The incident may be a recent trauma from which the client has been unable to recover or an old trauma that recent circumstances have triggered. In either case, basic TIR methodology is employed but some alteration might be needed where old traumas have been triggered.

Recent or Unresolved Traumas

These are traumas that have usually occurred in the past few days, weeks or months. The client has unremitting symptomatology from them. They remain unassimilated and are not integrated. Although these are occupying much of the client's attention, it is usually possible to complete the history assessment and time line before addressing them; occasionally it is not because the client is effectively still living through the incident and basic TIR is used at once.

Old Traumas

These are traumas presented as the present difficulty which have been recently triggered by some life event. They have been assimilated and accommodated to some degree or mental defences were rebuilt to contain them until something happened to reactivate them. Again, history-taking usually uncovers what has reactivated the trauma. Often this is simply a recent incident similar to the original one.

There are, however, some instances where a client presents an old incident as the identified source of current symptoms, and she is so immersed in it as to prevent history assessment or doing anything else except addressing this issue. In this instance, a counsellor might well simply address the incident with basic TIR.

WHAT HAS BEEN TRIGGERED VERSUS WHAT TRIGGERED IT

We have discussed this issue in part in the theory section in Chapter 2. Whether history-taking is done or not, if a client is presenting an incident which did not produce symptoms at the time and is now reactivated (e.g. producing symptoms or causing concerns), the counsellor is advised to discover what reactivated it before addressing it with TIR. There may be a more recent incident that needs looking at first and it might be crucial to address that. Without exploration, the client might not bring it up as it doesn't appear as a trauma. For example, a 40-year-old woman had an abortion 25 years ago and presents this as a source of great distress and wants to address it. The obvious thing to do is just that. Despite the client's attention on the incident, the counsellor explored how this incident had been triggered. It turned out that the client's daughter was pregnant, was considering an abortion and bringing up a lot of 'right to life' issues. These issues had not been so prevalent at the time of the client's abortion 25 years ago and she had not really considered them. The discussions with the daughter, not disturbing to the client or traumatic in themselves, had acted to reconstruct the client's trauma which she had easily recovered from at the time (e.g. she had not developed any symptoms that lasted beyond the period of a normal reaction). In the light of new information, new questions, the client was reconstruing her experience and feeling guilty, upset and ashamed. Although this incident still needed to be addressed with basic TIR, the client benefited from seeing it in the broader perspective. Seeing how it was triggered considerably changed how she viewed it.

Counsellors are advised wherever possible to establish what triggered an old trauma before using TIR with it. Sample questions for this exploration include: 'Has this trauma always bothered you?' 'Were there times when you felt OK about it?', 'Has anything occurred recently that made you think of it?', 'Are there any situations that you encounter that tend to trigger it?'

In the event of having utilized TIR to deal with an old trauma straight away, and the client has not identified triggers, then it is possible to do it afterwards. It is a matter of the counsellor's judgement as to whether this appears to be necessary.

BASIC TIR PROCEDURE

1. Address the client's presented incident whether it is a recent trauma or chosen by the client from his trauma list created from the assessment.
2. (If not already obvious.) Make sure that the client is interested in addressing the incident with TIR.
3. Establish when the incident took place. The purpose of this step is to locate the incident in time and orient the client to that time period. Sometimes the client will come up with an actual date such as '12 December 1996 at 2.30 a.m.'. Sometimes the client has only a vague idea and says 'a few years ago'. An exact date is not necessary but it is helpful to pin the incident down as far as possible using landmarks such as 'Do you recall where you were working at the time?' and 'When would that have been?' or 'How old was your son at the time?' or 'Was it winter, summer, spring, autumn?'. Use any pertinent question to help the client satisfy himself that he has roughly recognized when the incident took place. Do not badger the client for an exact time when he is unable to give one.

   Sometimes the question of *when* is more easily established by combining it with *where*.
4. Establish where the incident took place. Where was the client at the time? For example, 'I was sitting in class at Pembury Road school' or 'I was on safari somewhere in the Kenyan outback' or 'I was sitting in the front carriage of the Brighton to London train facing the front'.
5. Establish the beginning of the incident. What point marks the beginning of this trauma or experience? For example, 'I heard a scream' or 'I smelled burning' or 'I got the call from my mother'. Typically, clients will identify the point the incident first impacted on them rather than what the counsellor really wants to include, which is the prior normal experience and expectations that contrast with the trauma. This is

established by asking what the client was doing before that. For example, 'I was reading my book on the park bench' or 'I'd just come in from work and was having dinner'.

6. Establish the parameters of the incident. Find out from the client how long the incident lasted. With an incident such as a car accident, the client might say 'a few seconds'. The client might include police and ambulance intervention and say 'a few hours', or the client might even say 'It is still going on' (meaning the trauma is still there affecting him right up to the present). With the client, establish when the incident itself, rather than the experience of it, seemed to end. This would cover any period of shock, hospital treatment or other immediate consequences.

Again, do not badger the client for exact times. The counsellor just wants rough parameters that enable the client to see the incident as boundaried and not all enveloping. In the case of an incident consisting of multiple events over a long period of time (for example, being held hostage for several weeks), it might be necessary to break the incident into chunks – particularly if the client has difficulty confronting the whole experience. For example, following a car accident the client is in hospital for nine months having a series of operations including an amputation, and during this time discovers that his passenger has died and he has lost his job. Such an incident may need to be broken down into individual incidents and separately addressed. If this is done, then the client is invited to do it – the chunks may not be what the counsellor expects. For example, the client indicates that he can not deal with the whole nine months because it is too overwhelming. The counsellor proposes breaking it down into the sections described above, but the client disagrees. He states, 'The worst part was when I was transferred to the other hospital and was in traction for three months with no visitors. Then the amputation was another. The rest doesn't bother me so much.' If incidents need to be chunked, ask the client how *he* would break it down into phases or sections of the whole experience and then use each step of basic TIR to address each section. The client can be asked which piece he is interested in addressing first, next and so on until all the sections have been done. (If no full end point has been achieved, it might then be necessary to go through the whole to enable the client to tie it all together.)

7. Ask the client to place himself at the beginning of the incident (established on step 5).

8. Ask the client what he is aware of at that time. (Some clients find it easier to do this and the rest of the procedure with their eyes closed; others have no problem introspecting with their eyes open. The counsellor should give the client the option at this point.) For example, 'I am

aware of sitting in my seat on the train. I am engrossed in my book and the images I'm imagining from the story. I have no perception of what is going on in the carriage' or 'I'm aware of the taste of my food. My wife's conversation and then the phone ringing.'

9. Ask the client to go through the incident from that point, viewing all of it in sequence. (NB: The analogy of a videotape can be used here but it breaks down if it is interpreted to mean that the client is a spectator. Even when a client's trauma is a witnessed one – such as seeing someone killed by a train – he is still an actor, if only an 'extra', in that scene. Do not encourage clients to dissociate themselves from the event while engaging with it in the session.) The counsellor should remind the client before this step that he wants the client to tell him whatever should cross his mind during this process – for example, talking about his thoughts and feelings at the time of the incident – and his review of these things is part of the procedure rather than 'sticking to the story' of the incident.

On the first time through, the client should describe the incident as he experienced it. On subsequent passes, the counsellor may have the client review it silently and then tell him what happened. While the client is going through the incident, the counsellor does nothing except have his full attention on the client and acknowledge where appropriate. (Refer to the rules in Chapter 1 and the section on communication in Chapter 1. There are examples later in this chapter of violations of those rules.) There is no discussion, no reflecting back of the client's thoughts, feelings or experiences. Such actions only seem to distract the client. Quiet acknowledgements and the counsellor's full attention are all that are needed to support the client and ensure that he is being heard and comprehended.

10. When the client has finished going through the incident, the counsellor acknowledges him, allows the client to make any comment on it and then asks him to go back to the beginning and go through it again. (It is best to do this in two steps – having the client let you know when he has reached the beginning again.) This time the counsellor has the option of having the client review the incident silently and then tell him about it. This should be done when the counsellor is satisfied that the client is able to examine the incident in detail all the way through without the necessity to talk through its content while doing so. Having clients review an incident silently when they are able to do so is recommended as this is thought to permit processing unimpeded by the necessity to simultaneously articulate in language the content of the incident.

At no time should the counsellor discuss the incident, make comments or interpretations. He simply has the client review the incident as many times as needed to the point where it is discharged provided only that there is evidence that information processing is occurring. Such evidence can take the following form*:

- The client's recall or perception of the incident is changing in some way. Change is the most obvious signal that information processing is occurring.
- The client is becoming more relieved and there is evidence (body language, facial expression, verbal expression of change in emotion) that he is moving towards resolution.
- The client is manifesting an emotional discharge (such as crying or expressing anger).
- The client is becoming aware of new aspects of the incident – remembering details he had forgotten.
- The client is becoming able, or more able, to perceive the incident.
- The client is becoming more aware of the reactions he had and decisions he made at the time of the incident and is re-evaluating these.

11. If having been through the incident several times, none of the above is occurring and an end point has not been reached, then use any of the TIR additional questions (Chapter 8) that might be relevant to assist processing. If there is still no end point, then ask the client if there is an earlier related or connected incident and, if so, repeat the entire procedure on that incident. (NB. If there is a known sequence of related incidents, then it may take several sessions to address them. In this case, the counsellor should end a session at a comfortable point of session completion as possible. See Chapter 9, for suggestions on ending a session when resolution has not been reached.)

Sample questions for finding an earlier incident: 'Is there an earlier incident that relates to this one?' or 'Did this incident trigger an experience that has happened to you before?' or 'Is there an earlier incident that is connected to this one?' or 'Has anything similar to this ever happened to you before?' The counsellor wants the client to tell him whatever comes to mind when he asks this question – even if the connection is not obvious. For example, when asked about earlier related incidents, a client who had a road traffic accident recalled an image of an argument he had with his father five years previously. Once he had examined this earlier incident, it became obvious to him that the connection was the strong feelings of anger in both incidents.

---

* This list was adapted, with permission, from French and Gerbode (1995)

It is imperative that the counsellor does not interpret or evaluate whether or not it is appropriate to examine ANY incident a client brings up in response to this question – regardless of whether it makes sense to the counsellor or to the client. If an incident appears in response to this question, it should be examined. If the client is concerned because he cannot see immediately what the connection between the incidents is, the counsellor should reassure him and continue with the process. Remember that this method is process-oriented rather than content-oriented. How an earlier incident is connected with a later one often only emerges *after* it has been addressed. In many cases basic TIR on presented incidents goes to an end point without having to address earlier related incidents in the same session.

Look for Changes*

Change of any kind is what will tell the counsellor that he is on the right track in continuing to have the client review repeatedly a given incident. It can be change in the content of the incident, such as more or different characters appearing in the incident, the scene being described from a different viewpoint, the perception that 'It seems as though maybe George was actually behind the door . . . ', 'I'm actually not sure it was George that did it; maybe it was Greg!', or even 'I'm beginning to see how painful that actually was!' All such changes in the content tell the counsellor to continue reviewing the same incident.

On the other hand, the change the counsellor sees may not be in the story content but in the client's affect – the feelings that he demonstrates as he reviews the incident repeatedly. Thus, for example, though the story itself may remain relatively unchanged in successive reviews, he may begin by sounding and looking bored as he describes the incident . . . then become angry during another review . . . then overcome by grief in another . . . then rage . . . then boredom again, and so forth. The counsellor treats change in affect exactly as he treats change in content – he simply continues to have the client review the incident.

It may at first take several reviews of the incident – possibly even three or four – with little or no observable change occurring in either affect or content before the client begins to actually contact the charge contained in it.

---

* This section was adapted, with permission, from French and Gerbode (1995)

Earlier Incidents

Occasionally, where a sequence of incidents exists, the client's attention might shift from the incident being addressed to an earlier one. More often than not, it is because the later incident is discharged enough and the earlier one is now accessible and of greater interest. If this happens, the counsellor should simply switch to the earlier one and use the procedure with that. In rare instances, the client might try to switch attention to another incident because he is having trouble staying in contact with the existing one. In this instance, the counsellor would need to discover what problem the client is having with the incident being addressed and take the appropriate actions to help the client through it. A way of doing this is to chunk the incident. Have the client review what he can stay in contact with and incrementally have him contact bits of the whole until the incident is dealt with.*

The Importance of Repeatedly Reviewing the Incident†

When a person is permitted to review a painfully charged incident only once, one of two things can be the case. Either he will not really contact the incident and its charge, or he will become upset. In the first case, he will simply offer the counsellor a 'pre-packaged', 'sanitized', manageable version of the story, much as a person – even if he knew he was quite ill – might answer 'Fine' in response to a friend or stranger's cheery 'social' question, 'How are you?'. In the second case, he might plunge into the charge in the incident just as he has many times in the past. As a parallel to this phenomenon, consider the case of someone who is out for a social evening with friends for the first time since losing a much-loved spouse. He 'holds it together' almost well right up to the moment when someone comes up to him and says, 'I was so sorry to hear about your wife's death' – the trigger that brings the traumatic event into the present – at which point he begins to sob.

In neither of these circumstances may the client discover or resolve anything. In the first instance, nothing happens. In the second, he contacts the incident and becomes very upset . . . but by itself, that's simply something upsetting that has happened to him many times before. In short, he

---

* See Chapter 9 for remedies to this kind of situation.

† This section was adapted, with permission, from French and Gerbode (1995)

will not have been helped in either case. The evidence of lack of resolution is that he is seeking out counselling now, despite having talked about the experience once on a number of separate occasions.

BASIC TIR SUMMARY

Incident	The presented incident to be addressed.
Trigger	If an old incident, then how was it recently triggered?
Time	When did the incident occur?
Location	Where did the incident occur?
Beginning	When did the incident start? What was happening just before that?
Perception	What was the client aware of at the start of the incident?
Process	Have the client go through the incident, describing it in detail – with anything else that occurs to him while he is doing this.
Repeat process	Have the client review the incident as many times as needed silently and then tell you what happened until an end point.
Additional questions	If no end point occurs, use additional questions as needed.
Earlier incident	If still no end point occurs, ask for an earlier related incident(s) and apply basic TIR as above.

A REVIEW OF THE END POINT

In Chapter 1 we listed the criteria for an end point. In Chapter 6 we discussed these criteria in more depth when referring to Unblocking. Here we list them with some further explanation and cover how the counsellor can check with the client to see if resolution has been achieved.

As we said in Chapter 1, the end point criteria are the guide for the counsellor as to when to end a session – illustrating that the client is resolving the incident. The end point is a process measure rather than a content one – e.g. the counsellor is observing the process, not evaluating the significance or meaning of what the client is saying. By definition, resolution involves feeling more positive about the experience, feeling that the experience has now been put to rest, so the evidence the counsellor observes should be in the direction of being more positive in order for the counsellor to consider that an end point has occurred.

From Chapter 1, the criteria include:

1. Change in the client's emotional state in a positive direction (preferably strongly positive direction). This includes:
   - A return of normal colour to the face.
   - The client is laughing, smiling or demonstrating that he is feeling better.
   - The client makes statements illustrating that he is feeling better or feeling positive emotions such as feeling peaceful, feeling happy; the trauma has lost its intensity and no longer feels important.
   - The client's body position indicates a more relaxed internal state.
   - The client reports that negative physical sensations have disappeared.

2. The client's attention shifts from concentrating on his mental environment to an awareness of the external environment:
   - The client makes sustained eye contact with the counsellor.
   - The client notices things in the room.
   - The client is attracted by things in the physical environment (including feeling hungry, noticing the time, noticing external noises).
   - The client comments on activities he will be involved in after the session (e.g. he is going to the gym after session, must make a call, has a meeting).
   - The client comments on the counsellor or something about the counsellor.

3. There is evidence of a cognitive shift – the client's thinking about the meaning of the traumatic experience has changed.
   - The client states that he has achieved insight into the experience.
   - The client reframes the traumatic experience in terms of how it represents a learning experience.
   - The client makes connections between the trauma and other experiences in his life.
   - The client reports that the trauma feels finished and is no longer as significant.
   - The client reports that the experience now makes sense and talks about its meaning to him.
   - The client loses interest in the trauma and in talking about the trauma.
   - The client feels the trauma is now a historical, past event rather than in the present.

Ideally, the counsellor wants to see some evidence of all three points to be present before ending the TIR session. Sometimes, the evidence is very observable and the counsellor need not seek too much confirmation from the client before ending the session. However, at other times, it can be very difficult for the counsellor to assess through observation alone where the client is in this process. In the case when the evidence is very observable, the counsellor may choose only to ask the client how the incident or area seems at the present time. Often, the client will respond by giving more information on the cognitive shift he has experienced and any insights that he has achieved. At this point, it would be appropriate to end the session.

When communicating with others who use TIR (either on session notes for supervision or in supervisory conversations), we tend to use a type of short-hand to discuss where the client is in the process. When the client meets the criteria for the points above, we describe the client as having 'positive indicators'. If the client is demonstrating evidence of emotional charge we describe this as having 'negative indicators'. This short-hand works well once a counsellor is very clear what evidence of an end point looks like; however, initially at least, it is always best to describe the evidence the counsellor has observed.

In cases where the counsellor is unsure of where the client is in the process, there are a variety of questions he can ask to assess what to do next. He can ask the client how the incident or area seems at present. If the client reports that it is still upsetting or confusing in any way, the counsellor has the client continue with basic TIR procedure. Alternatively, the counsellor could ask one of the additional questions in the next chapter and then continue the basic TIR procedure.

When using basic TIR procedure, an end point is usually achieved addressing the presented incident. Where there is a sequence of incidents, or earlier incidents triggered by the current one, then only by moving down and addressing the earlier incidents can an end point be achieved. The problem for the counsellor is that when addressing a presented incident, he has no real idea of the extent to which the charge contained in it is a result of previous connected incidents. Charge from earlier incidents may have been transferred to the present one – especially when the client is unaware of previous incidents having been triggered. A clue that this is happening is that the incident being addressed has been reviewed several times, with additional questions used, and is yet not discharging. It is at this point that the counsellor asks for earlier related incidents. However, sometimes a counsellor might well be unsure about the status of the incident – whether it is discharging or actually becoming more charged due to earlier connected incidents. In this case he should enquire: 'How does the incident seem to you at this moment?', 'Is it lightening up?', 'Does it seem to be discharging or remaining the same?' When incidents are not discharging, and are getting harder (heavier) to look at instead of easier (lighter), then earlier connected incidents should be asked for and addressed.

Some of the additional questions in the following chapter can be used to help the client to articulate a cognitive shift – or to help the counsellor check to see if a cognitive shift has occurred. Sometimes the client does not articulate the insight he achieves following the cognitive shift in the same session. In this case, the counsellor will usually find out more about the insight at the beginning of the next session when he asks the client how things have been since the previous session.

TWO EXAMPLES OF BASIC TIR SESSIONS

Here we present transcripts from each of the clients we are following throughout the book. The counsellor's statements are written in regular print and the client's statements are written in *italics*. Please note that in some cases, the counsellor has asked additional questions because he has observed something and the incident has stopped changing without an end point being achieved. In all cases, the observations of the counsellor are included in brackets and in regular print.

Mary's Session: Basic TIR on an Incident when her Father tried to Kill Her

(Mary was asked to pick the incident from her trauma list that she was most interested in.)

When my father tried to kill me. (Looks upset, is fidgeting.)

OK. Has this incident always bothered you?

Yes. I have had intrusive thoughts about it and nightmares about it and it was brought to mind when we did the history.

All right. When did it happen?

When I was 15 years old.

Yes. Where did the incident occur?

We were in my father's pub.

Fine. How long did the incident last?

I'm not sure, probably just a few minutes.

OK. When did the incident start?

When my father became angry.

OK. What was happening just before that?

It was the staff Christmas party and my father was drinking. That's where it starts really.

Fine. Close your eyes and place yourself at the beginning of the incident.

OK.

What are you aware of?

My father, a big pub size bottle of red wine. My father's red angry face.

OK. Move through the incident in sequence with as much detail as possible. (Mary silently reviews the incident. As she does, she begins to cry. Then she opens her eyes.) All right. Please tell me what happened.

There was a staff Christmas party and my father was drinking. He was being angry and everyone pretended not to notice but we were all aware of it. We were near the juke box. Jeannie, a friend, was there and her husband, Ralph, was dancing with a woman who has just left her own husband. Jeannie is upset so I cut in so that she doesn't get more upset. Her husband is a good dancer and it is fun to dance with him. My father is watching me. I can feel it and decide to continue anyway because it is fun. (Mary's body is very rigid, she is shaking.) *Next he says to take my sister home. She is 5 years old and doesn't want to go home. She's crying and I know if he hears her he will hit me so I hit her to stop.* (Mary is crying.) *She cries even louder. He comes out shouting 'you whore'. All of the staff hear and I am ashamed and embarrassed. I call him a fucking bastard and I run home. I can't go back in the room. So I go to bed. My other sister has the tape recorder playing something. My father comes running into the room and grabs me by the throat squeezing hard.* (Mary is speaking in a frightened tone of voice and very rapidly.) *My mother comes in and is banging on his back. He pushes her away and she leaves and then he leaves. My 5-year-old sister is crying and it's all my fault.*

(Making eye contact, and said in a firm, compassionate voice.) Got it. Please go back to the beginning of the incident.

OK. (Mary closes her eyes again.)

Good. Move through the incident in sequence until you reach the end. (Mary silently reviews the incident then opens her eyes and looks at the counsellor.) OK. Please tell me what happened.

(Mary sighs.) *I'm talking with Jeannie about this guy I fancy called Mark. My father is aware we are into each other. He's a drummer in a band. My father told him if he comes near me he will shoot his balls off. He did this in front of people. I know Mark won't come near me now. The next part is the same as the first time. When my father is watching me I feel really trapped.* (Mary repeats the body of the story. Her tone is angry this time.) *When my father came into the room, he grabbed the tape recorder and threw it across the room and pushed my sister before he grabbed me by the throat and started squeezing. I'm thinking 'This is it. I'm going to die.' I don't even feel like fighting. It has been such a long time and he hates me.* (Mary is crying.) *That's a stupid thing to say to somebody.* (She tells the rest of the story – with the same content as last time.)

All right. Please go back to the beginning of the incident.

OK. It's like it doesn't matter who else is there. He just gets angry and shows it. The red wine is always a bad sign. I don't care anymore, why bother. It doesn't matter. It feels weird. Everybody else is a cardboard cut-out this time – just me and my father. The only thing that matters or stands out is when he calls me a whore. This time he has gone to far. I see myself hitting my sister because I'm feeling desperate because he'll hit me. (The story is the same). *I cannot feel the impact of my mother's blows on his back. He's going to hit my sister – shit she is only 5! Already she thinks this stuff is her fault. I can't understand how my mother could sleep with my father after this. So I go to sleep. Nobody talks to my father the next day and he says he can't understand why no one is speaking to him. He says he didn't do anything wrong. We all just look at each other. Mother says very cuttingly – it's very convenient isn't it. My sister goes missing and we find her on the road. She says she wants to run away.*

Got it. Please go back to the beginning of the incident.

Yes. (Mary closes her eyes.)

Thanks. Move through the incident in sequence until you reach the end.

There was a Hot Chocolate song on the juke box. People had tried to get my father to dance – there were more than 20 people there. He won't dance. I know he's watching me – he's always been watching me – ever since I can remember. (The story is the same as the last time. Mary is speaking in a more matter of fact tone.) *My middle sister always tries to keep the peace – but this time she cannot.* (The rest of the story is the same – no changes and it appears to have levelled out.)

OK. Is this incident getting easier to review or harder to review?

The part with my father is somewhat lighter. My mother's responsibility in this still feels very significant and heavy – typical of my mother.

All right. Is there a related earlier incident?

Yes. It was the year earlier. I can see my father going out the door.

Fine. Place yourself at the beginning of the incident.

OK. (Mary closes her eyes.)

Move through the incident in sequence with as much detail as possible. (Mary examines it silently and then opens her eyes.) All right. Please tell me what happened.

My mother left my father and brought the three of us to some house – grand-mother's house. Father was at the door. Grandma doesn't know what to do – he is being very nice to her so she let's him in. My uncle is out back with a hammer. He's really angry with my father. Father apologies to mother and says he wants to speak to her. My mother says she doesn't know what to do. Ten minutes later my uncle comes in and says he'll kill the bastard. (Mary reviews this incident five more times with significant changes in content and affect. The incident has levelled off but no end point has been reached.)

Did you decide or conclude anything at that time?

That things were a waste of time. I should play dead. I cannot have a mother and remember this – that she goes back to him no matter what he does to us. The only way I can have a mother is to pretend it is all a dream. (Mary is looking calmer but there is still no end point. She requests a break because she is very hungry. A break for lunch is taken at this point. The session is resumed after lunch.)

Is there a related earlier incident?

Yes. I was 2 or 3 years old. It lasted about half an hour. I can see my father coming home from work.

OK. Place yourself at the beginning of the incident. (Mary closes her eyes and nods yes.) Fine. Move through the incident in sequence until you reach the end. (Mary silently reviews the incident.) Good. Please tell me what happened.

Father came home from work wearing his work clothes. I am in the middle of the floor – I have ankle boots with a ribbon on, a cardigan and a skirt. My mother is holding the baby and there are toys everywhere. Father doesn't like toys every-where. He saying something and his hands are going like this. (Mary demon-strates with her hands – her father is pointing angrily.) *Mother says something. He says she has to learn sometime. I am dragged upstairs holding on to the banister. Not saying anything. To my room. He closes the door and locks it. Takes off his belt with the big buckle on it. He's hitting me with the belt – with the buckle end. I'm up on the ceiling watching him – it doesn't feel real – it feels like someone else. He's hitting her all over her body – her head snaps back before he catches her with the buckle on her head – it's bleeding. Mother comes upstairs with the baby and puts the baby on the bed. He freezes. She says* 'see what you've done' and sends him to the bathroom for the medicine box. They put a bandage on my head to hold until it stops bleeding. The next day a neighbour asks what happened to the child and my mother says I cut my head on the play pen. That's it.

(The second time through this incident, Mary does not watch from the ceiling. She is feeling the pain and quite upset. The third time through the incident, the story is the same and Mary says it feels somehow unimportant. The fourth time through the incident she reports feeling still and calm. She then says the following.) My mother didn't protect me or couldn't protect me. I decided that she was not trustworthy. There are more incidents connected with my mother but they are not connected to this group of incidents. I feel these are finished – she couldn't guard or protect me. (Mary laughs.) It's no wonder I've always had problems trusting. I'd like to look at the other stuff with my mother in another session. This feels done now. (Mary was looking better – her body posture was relaxed, her face was normal colour rather than flushed or drained of colour, she was reporting feeling calm and relaxed and there was evidence of a cognitive shift and new insight.)

Got it. Is there anything you want to add before we end the session?

No. That feels a good place to stop. The other stuff is separate and I know we will get to it eventually. I'm looking forward to a nice hot meal when I get home.

(End of excerpt.)

Renee's Session: Basic TIR on an Incident in which she was Mugged in 1979

(Renee was asked to pick an incident from her trauma list that she was interested in examining. She picked this incident when she was mugged in 1979.)

When in 1979 did this happen?

I think it was October. What led up to it was we lived in Brixton on an estate. Roger was working for a shop-fitting firm. I was at home and the phone went. I had got in at 2-ish. A woman, a nurse, said Roger had an accident – fallen off a ladder. He was going to hospital. I got the kids ready when they came home from school. Roger had brought a girl home two weeks before. He took her out but he didn't come home until the next day. He had lipstick all over his shirt. Two weeks later was the accident. I think she might have had something to do with it. We went to the hospital to see him. He was sedated anyway. I thought there must be more to it. I was dropped off and walked back onto the estate. It was a bit dark.

I had my bag on my shoulder. I was being pulled backwards downstairs and my bag was being pulled off. I went berserk and went after them. They got away. Roger called from the hospital. I cried. The bag was found empty. I got a few phone calls that were very funny. Got frightened by it. Didn't go into the stairwells again and didn't go out in the dark. When I think about it, it could have been worse. Could have been banged up. It hasn't happened since. Now I keep money in my jeans. I have to think about things like that. Mostly I drive now. I was already in a depressed state. (Renee laughs.) *The whole marriage I was depressed. It was part of the pattern – Roger's drinking, his girlfriend, later the suicide. It was all part of that. I felt insecure, unloved and then the mugging. Roger always denied ever going with another woman. I was a drudge at the time. He wouldn't let me wear makeup. I never had my hair done and that depressed me.* (Renee laughs.) *The young girl was dressed up and made up. I don't know why I made dinner for them. Must have been something wrong with me. I'll never get to the bottom of it. I said to him the other day it doesn't affect me anymore what he says and does. He was so uncaring and unfeeling.*

All right. Please go back to the beginning of the incident.

OK.

Fine. Please go through it again step by step.

I got mugged, broke down and cried. I called the police. They asked me to describe the mugger – I said 'black' – that's all I knew. I was very frightened. I didn't know whether I'd be banged up. The kids screamed. I was angry at the neighbour who didn't come out. I just stayed indoors for two days and called into work saying I was sick. I went to visit Roger at the weekend. He said don't cry about it. I just carried on. I just bounce back. (Renee reviews the incident again with no change in affect or content. The first time through the incident, she was speaking in an angry and upset tone. This time through the incident, she was speaking conversationally.)

I think I see that. Did you decide or conclude anything at that time?

I made myself more aware. Now I always turn round if I hear anyone behind me. I never wear jewellery and I don't carry anything of any real value. Always put keys in my pocket. I didn't trust. I was anxious for a little while. I had the depression already. I got to the stage where I didn't want to go out to work.

OK. How does it seem at the moment?

I don't get any sense of the fear now. I found out later that the mugger was a member of [a pop group]. I saw them on telly years later and I would get the hump. (Renee laughs.) *If it was him I hope he thinks about it from time to time. I can think about it now. I can see it but it doesn't want to make me cry. I don't feel sad and it doesn't effect me anymore.*

(The session was ended here. Renee was laughing, looking more relaxed in body posture, stating that the incident was no longer a problem and making connections between the incident and the rest of her mental state at the time. Renee examined the other incidents briefly mentioned during this one in separate sessions.)

(End of excerpt.)

ADDRESSING A CLIENT'S CONCERNS DURING A TIR SESSION

Though the rules for TIR and related methods suggest that the counsellor relies solely on placing his full attention on the client, staying in emotional contact with the client, asking questions and acknowledging responses during the course of the TIR session, there are occasions where the counsellor must step outside the rules. The primary occasion when this is true is when the client brings up a concern that needs to be addressed during the session. In this case, a concern refers to any time a client raises an issue that requires action on the part of the counsellor. Here are some examples of concerns: 'I have to go to the bathroom', 'I'm hungry', 'I must make a phone call by 3 p.m.', 'I'm bored with this', 'I have a headache'.

Certain concerns require actual physical action – for example, if the client states he needs to use the bathroom, the counsellor must respond by taking a break in the session. Other concerns require further information before it can be determined if action needs to be taken (such as a session break or ending the session) or if continuing the session is likely to resolve the issue: 'I'm bored with this' and 'I have a headache' are examples of this type of concern. The first thing the counsellor must find out when a concern of this type is raised is when the feeling or discomfort began. Headaches that begin in session are sometimes a specific phenomenon and are addressed in Chapter 9. Other physical complaints (and emotional responses) that begin during a session are usually best addressed by continuing the session. As we discussed earlier, often during TIR the client will experience the physical sensations he had at the time of the trauma – therefore, continuing with TIR until these are defused is usually the best remedy in these situations. We mention this during the client education and remind clients of this education if these issues arise in session. Boredom is also a specific phenomenon which is covered in Chapter 9.

Examples of Concerns Raised in Session

In the example of basic TIR taken from Mary's work earlier in this chapter, there is an example of hunger being raised as a concern during a long session in which she examined multiple incidents. The incident had been defused but was not resolved, and it was clear there was an earlier connected incident when Mary brought up the fact that she was hungry. The session had already been in progress for two hours by this point and it was past lunch time. The counsellor decided at that point to end the session for a lunch break. Before doing this, she checked with Mary to make sure that she felt grounded enough for a break. Mary agreed that this was fine and the TIR was started again after lunch.

The following is an excerpt from a session with Jane in which she was examining a serious road traffic accident. On the fourth review, Jane was in the midst of telling the story when she grimaced.

I don't remember feeling like this during the incident. The pain in my leg is horrific. I must have felt it during the incident. My leg was crushed. It really hurts.

OK. When did you start feeling this pain?

Just a few minutes ago. (There are tears running down Jane's face.)

I've got it. Remember when we talked during education about feeling the physical pain from the incident during TIR?

Yes. You said it was possible. I didn't think it would be this intense.

OK. I realize it is very intense but if you can manage the pain for a while longer, it should stop. Usually continuing the TIR procedure is the best remedy in this situation – as the pain is coming from the incident – and once it is integrated it will stop.

I remember you saying that. I can manage it. (Jane continued TIR and reviewed the incident twice more. As she didn't mention the pain and her face relaxed, the counsellor checked to see if this had shifted.)

Are you still feeling the pain in your leg?

No, actually it's gone now. (Jane was smiling and the session continued.)

(End of transcript.)

If the client feels safe enough and can feel that the counsellor has his full attention on her, she will usually be willing to continue through the worst part of the incident until it begins to defuse and the charge is reduced. If the counsellor is unsure of himself, the client will find it hard to feel safe and it will be difficult to continue through the worst part of the session.

THEMATIC TIR

Thematic TIR is a TIR application used where there is either no presented incident or when an incident (that has been addressed) has triggered or revealed 'themes' that might have roots in other incidents. A theme can be described as the client's statement of an unwanted condition such as an attitude, idea, emotional reaction, feeling or sensation. It is called a theme because it is characteristic in a sequence of traumatic experiences. For example 'a fear of public speaking' might be a specific fear a client identifies during the assessment. With this example, the counsellor might find a sequence of traumatic experiences such as: hosting a birthday party at which he had to speak; being best man at a wedding; attending a support group; speaking at a local council meeting; having to take part in a school play; being made to read aloud in primary school. The fear of public speaking is a theme that connects this sequence of traumatic experiences. These incidents themselves most likely would not have emerged during the history-taking but the theme does, and it is that which enables the counsellor to access them using thematic TIR.

A complex traumatic incident might contain a number of themes which become highlighted by the incident and remain inadequately addressed during basic TIR. For example, the incident 'the death of my wife' might contain and highlight several themes very familiar to the client which may need to be specifically addressed, such as the attitude 'Life is futile', the emotional reaction 'uncontrollable grief', 'a sensation of numbness', 'a feeling of isolation'. Such items may have their own sequences of incidents and root incident. For example, the attitude 'Life is futile' may have a sequence something like this:

Death of my wife (the recent incident)
Death of father
Death of grandmother
Loss of job
Failure in exams
Failure at a sporting event at school
Being spanked by mother (the root)

There is no suggestion that themes addressed with TIR will simply vanish as a result. Some of a client's themes may be based on physiology, others may require a variety of psychological interventions. 'Fear of public speaking', for example, when addressed with thematic TIR, should reduce the accumulation of emotional and cognitive charge that has been encapsulated in those incidents and provide some insight into the difficulty. If the client is motivated to fully deal with the fear, he will probably need to join 'Toastmasters' or some other group to practise the skill which allows the condition to be resolved. If thematic TIR is used to address a 'feeling of isolation', then again charge should be removed and insight gained, but if the client is deficient in social skills or marginalized in his community then other interventions will obviously be needed.

Counsellors can use thematic TIR in two ways:

1. To continue to address a severe traumatic incident that warrants further attention. This is done by asking the client for attitudes, emotional reactions, ideas, feelings or sensations connected with the incident and examining any the client is interested in.
2. To address themes that the client has brought up during the history stage or in other sessions. This would normally be done after the client's list of presented traumas has been addressed with basic TIR. A list can be compiled of the client's themes and the client asked to pick out any he would like to address with TIR. This could be a separate list compiled from the history and subsequent sessions.

Thematic TIR has slightly different instructions for the client, which are as follows: Having found a theme the client is interested in addressing, the counsellor asks him to find an incident that contains (that theme). The counsellor should insert the client's wording of the theme in his instruction.

Unlike basic TIR where, in many cases, resolution is reached without addressing earlier related incidents, in thematic TIR the counsellor expects to encounter a sequence of incidents. This is because a theme, by definition, is something common to a number of incidents. Incidents found would be addressed using the same procedure as with basic TIR except that, as soon as the counsellor feels the client has processed the incident being addressed (which is when it stops changing and might occur only after a couple of reviews), the counsellor would ask for an earlier incident containing (the theme).

Counsellors are advised to beware of assuming that themes will inevitably go back to childhood, 'the womb' or even a 'past life existence'. The counsellor is looking for an end point: evidence of reduction in emotional or cognitive charge and an insight or cognitive shift. This might occur in a more recent incident or a very early incident. In any event, the session is ended when an end point occurs. (As a reminder, see the section on end points earlier in this chapter.)

In thematic TIR, it is much more likely that, when addressing a later incident, the client's attention will shift to an earlier one. If this occurs, then the counsellor can assume that sufficient charge was removed from the later one to enable the client to look at the earlier incident. In this case, immediately switch to the earlier incident.

There have been times (rarely) when addressing an incident that a client identifies a later incident in a sequence and his attention moves to that. If this happens, follow the client's attention and address the later one, coming back to the earlier one as necessary. The important thing is, as with any TIR, the counsellor must keep the client on the subject he is addressing whether it is a presented incident or a theme. The structure of TIR is geared to assessing and compartmentalizing different issues the client has, and addressing them piecemeal. A client finds stability and safety with this approach, which can be ruined if a counsellor allows him to wander all over his trauma network triggering everything and discharging nothing. (NB. If a client is finding more interest in other incidents or themes that the counsellor is not addressing, there may be something wrong with the counsellor's assessment or he may have overlooked an end point on what he is doing. See Chapter 9 for more on this issue and obtain supervision as needed.)

Case Example of a Thematic TIR Session

Here we present a transcript from Mary. The counsellor's statements are written in regular print and the client's statements are written in *italics*. Please note that in some cases, the counsellor has asked additional questions because she has observed something and the incident has stopped changing without an end point being achieved. In all cases, the observations of the counsellor are included in brackets and in regular print.

The Theme: 'Feeling Like I am in a Glass Bubble'

Please find an incident that contains the feeling that you are in a glass bubble.

OK. It was during my second year of university – when I was 18 years old.

OK. How long did the incident last?

About three weeks. I'm not sure exactly.

Fine. Where were you at the time?

In a glass bubble! (Mary laughs.) *At university – don't get anything more precise.*

OK. Have you found the beginning of the incident?

Yes. I'm there.

Fine. Move through the incident step by step until you reach the end. (Mary goes through the incident silently and then opens her eyes.) OK. Please tell me what happened.

I can't remember much. Josh was wearing an Aran jumper and jeans. There was a student boycott of the catering. I was more involved than he was. I think we went to a friend's flat – we were all from the same area. There was music playing. They don't really accept me. The girls' room was partitioned – one came in and was lying on her bed. I didn't see anything at first because Josh and I were kissing. She went out of the room and I don't remember anything else until we woke up one morning. He asked how I was and I said I was really tired. I asked how I got here and he said he brought me here. Told me not to worry. We were at his mother's house and went down to the kitchen. His mother was there and said hello. I didn't really remember meeting her but obviously had. He had no idea that I had been gone – in this glass bubble. (Mary is upset, shaking.)

OK. Please go back to the start of the incident.

OK.

Fine. Please move through it again, step by step until you reach the end. (Mary starts talking this time, rather than reviewing it silently.)

Josh and I were in this girl's flat. I was nervous – weird people were there. We drank a lot. Josh was rowdy. We were in the bedroom kissing. Jane came in and was not pleased so we left. I can remember the music that was on – Jim Croce, then Joan Armatrading. I wake up and am not sure where I was. Everybody was acting strangely. (Mary talks through the incident twice more with no change in content or affect.)

OK. Please find an earlier incident that contains the feeling that you are in a glass bubble.

OK. When I was 10 and someone was shouting at me.

Fine. How long did this incident last?

20 minutes and I was at school and it was the teacher shouting.

OK. Please place yourself at the beginning of that incident.

Yes. I fell asleep in class. We had been doing maths.

OK. Please move through the incident step by step until you reach the end. (Mary reviews the incident silently, then opens her eyes and begins to speak.)

I was in class – and we were doing maths and I was tired. I fell asleep and the teacher was shouting at me – then all of a sudden I was in the hall and going to my next class. It bothers me that I cannot remember the bit where I am in the glass bubble – that's how I feel then. But I can't connect with that bit of the story. (Mary looks concerned, a bit agitated.)

OK. Let's go through it again and see if you connect with that bit.

Fine. (Mary closes her eyes and reviews the incident silently. She then opens her eyes and begins to speak.) *It's no different, I don't want to move on if I can't remember.*

OK. I'm going to ask you a few questions and I'd like you to tell me whatever comes to mind as usual when we do this type of work. OK? (Said in soothing even tone of voice.)

Fine. (Mary takes a deep breath and relaxes her body position in the chair.)

OK. **When you have this feeling – where are you?**

Absent, nobody is home.

OK. **So who or what part of you is acting and speaking during this absence?**

Me. (Mary looks relieved, body posture relaxes further.) *The memory part is absent – but I am there. I can connect with the memory if I am willing to feel the pain of the incident – this is a way I used to cope. Now that I am willing to connect with the memory – it doesn't feel so important – I've managed intense pain when I have reviewed other memories and come out of it – so I know I could manage these memories. In fact, they aren't that intense – the other stuff we have looked at is much worse. I guess the reason this theme came up is because it is an old coping strategy that upset me – the memories or the actual incidents that prompted me to enter the glass bubble have been dealt with in TIR already – I was just concerned I would use this strategy again – when under stress and I don't like the feeling of being in a glass bubble – and losing the memory of a period of time. Intellectually, I know this is dissociation and it was a very useful strategy at the time. It is not useful now – I can cope – always have been able to – and can remain present and in contact while coping and get through things. My past will not repeat – so its a remnant of being a child who couldn't protect herself. I'm an adult now and can protect myself and manage my feelings – however intense.* (Mary is speaking in an animated tone – smiling, body posture relaxed.)

OK. How does this theme feel now?

Fine. It wasn't the theme that was charged really – it was the other stuff we have looked at – the feeling was really a way of coping rather than a theme in itself.

I feel confident now that I have new skills. And also, if this were to happen again – I would know what was happening – it wouldn't be automatic and I could stay in some kind of contact rather than feeling like I was in a glass bubble.

OK. Is there anything you wish to add before we end this session?

No. That's fine. (The session was ended here.)

(End of excerpt.)

VIOLATING THE RULES FOR TIR AND RELATED METHODS

Throughout the book, we have emphasized the importance of following the specific rules for using TIR and related methods as well as the specific communication style employed in these methods. As we discussed, these rules and style of communication help form the structure that creates the safety necessary for the client to examine painful traumatic material. Here we present some examples of violations of these rules from actual client sessions to once again illustrate the importance of this point. The client's comments are in *italics* and the counsellor's comments are in regular print.

Reflection Instead of Acknowledgement

During a session with Jeffrey, a newly trained counsellor using TIR decided to reflect back the client's thoughts instead of using a short acknowledgement. At this point in the session, Jeffrey was talking about his awareness of God.

It's like a pervasive feeling – of being loved, of being outside yourself. I don't experience God as being like a human being – it's more of a presence.

You see God as an all encompassing being?

No – pervasive – more of a feeling than a being – like I said, a presence.

OK. Let me see if I understand this, you see God as a presence, that is encompassing – not like a human presence?

No. Not really. I don't think of human beings in terms of presence. (A discussion of terminology ensued that continued for the next 10 minutes with the counsellor reflecting and the client correcting.)

I've lost the thread of the incident and what I was working on. (Jeffrey's tone of voice indicates frustration.)

OK. Let's find the beginning of the incident again.

(End of transcript.)

The session continued but no end point was reached. Jeffrey reported that he found it difficult to contact the incident again. In supervision, the error was pointed out and the supervisor suggested that the error would not have been so bad if a 10-minute discussion hadn't ensued and if the counsellor (having indulged in the discussion) had apologized and taken responsibility for Jeffrey losing the thread of the session. In the following session, Jeffrey was wary as he expressed to the counsellor that he now felt she didn't understand him. The counsellor apologized and after a session working on their relationship – the TIR counselling continued.

Interpreting the Client's Material – in the TIR Session

During a TIR workshop, a student was conducting an Unblocking session with another student on real material (as is usual practice). The Unblocking was about her relationship with her boyfriend. As she was discussing her insights just before the end of the session, the counsellor interpreted her material.

My problems with him are related to my view of men – mostly developed as a result of one major previous relationship where I got really hurt. Harold isn't really like Martin – so I can let go of those views. (The client is smiling and looking quite relaxed.)

You mentioned earlier in the workshop that you have problems with your father. Isn't it possible that your view of men was developed as a result of your relationship with your father?

That's a separate issue. (The client's tone of voice indicates anger and her expression is an angry one.) *What does a comment I made in passing earlier in the workshop have to do with this session anyway? And who are you to interpret things for me – particularly with a Freudian interpretation?!*

Well – if the shoe fits . . .

Get lost! (The client gets up and leaves the room.)

(End of transcript.)

In this case, the instructor spoke with the client and gained her agreement to fix the session in front of the student counsellor. This went very well and the student counsellor apologized to the client. It is likely that the client's reaction was more extreme in this situation than it would have been in a true counselling setting because the agreement between students on a workshop is quite different from the agreement between client and counsellor in a professional setting. However, clients do react with anger when they have been told their material will not be interpreted and the counsellor interprets it anyway.

Interpreting the Client's Material – Later in the Counselling

Audrey incorporated TIR into her practice and was using it with Joe in the course of some longer term analytic therapy. She educated Joe about the rules for TIR and related techniques and Joe agreed that it would be useful to use this method with some specific traumatic experiences. Prior to starting TIR, she decided to use Unblocking on their previous counselling relationship. During the Unblocking session, Joe disclosed that he found many of her interpretations and suggestions quite arrogant and patronizing. The session went well and Joe was very happy with the outcome. During the following three sessions, Audrey used TIR with Joe on specific traumatic material. Once that was complete, they returned to their more analytic relationship.

During the first session after they completed TIR, Audrey raised the issue of their relationship – bringing up the specific comments made by Joe during the Unblocking. Joe became quite angry and hurt and responded as follows:

First of all, you have broken your promise to me. I feel as if you are accusing me – making me feel bad because of what I said during that session when you said that I was supposed to tell you whatever came to mind and that you wouldn't react or interpret. You have interpreted – and judged me. I was so relieved during that session to be able to say all the things I had never mentioned and your response during the session was so accepting that I felt those issues were resolved and felt that in future I would be able to confront issues as they arose because I felt safe. Now, not only are you bringing up dead issues but you are violating our agreement. I don't think I can continue until we sort this out.

(End of transcript.)

In this case, Audrey was unwilling to move from her position that this material had a deeper meaning in terms of their relationship (transference) and that the material was still live for Joe. She insisted that Joe's feelings of betrayal and anger were related to other issues and not specific to her behaviour in this situation. Joe chose to end his therapy at this point. Six months after the therapy ended, Audrey brought these session tapes to TIR supervision.

It is important to note that the client in the previous example was most upset because the counsellor had violated the agreement they had made that she would not interpret the material he brought up in the TIR sessions. If a counsellor who uses interpretation wishes to integrate TIR into her practice, the best results will occur if the TIR rules are followed, even if this means that some of the material the client brings up is off limits for interpretation.

The next chapter covers the additional questions which a counsellor might find necessary when an incident or theme is not resolving.

8

USE OF ADDITIONAL QUESTIONS

In the previous chapter we covered the basic TIR and thematic TIR instructions. In this chapter we cover the additional questions that can be used during either type of TIR session when the incident is not changing or a client is not covering a particular facet of the trauma (e.g. there is emotion present but the client does not mention the cognitive content of the incident).

TIR is essentially a person-focused approach to enabling an individual to process, assimilate and accommodate the trauma he has experienced. As mentioned previously, although many traumas may appear to be broadly similar in impact, such as a car accident or bereavement, they always occur in individual, unique circumstances to a unique person. The understanding necessary to process the incident can therefore only be achieved by the individual who is aware of sufficient information necessary to resolve that particular incident. The counsellor obviously has no inside insight and is not in a position to correctly identify and interpret the significant elements contained within the client's experience. Furthermore, any interpretations made by the counsellor with his authority may inhibit the client's own insight by weighting importance on what the counsellor thinks is significant and drawing the client's attention to that rather than allowing him to view his experiences unhindered.

Any and all counsellor questions have the liability of containing a suggestion, because of either the language used or the pitch, tone, inflection or non-verbal communication that might accompany it. Ideally, TIR is conducted with a minimum of additional questions. In its 'pure' form the procedure enables the client to access and view the qualia of the experience and process it to the point of a resolution without any further counsellor interventions. However, whereas the ability to self-reflect and process information with a view to resolving internal as well as external information seems to be universal (excluding, perhaps, those with severe mental illness or learning disabilities), the degree to which this ability has been exercised by any individual seems to vary quite considerably. We use the terms 'cognitive literacy' and 'emotional literacy', which can be defined as the individual's ability to view or experience and then articulate either his thoughts or his emotions. Individuals well practised at viewing and processing information in their own mental environment may have become so as a result of engaging in previous therapy or for some other experiential or characterological reason. With these individuals, the 'pure' form of TIR is usually all that is needed. Such people will engage with their trauma in TIR and be able to view and articulate the images, cognitions and emotions that comprise it. They will be able to make connections along the lines of their own traumatic associative networks and arrive at a point of resolution without any further direction on the part of the counsellor.

Not surprisingly, we have observed that the self-reflective and analytical demands placed upon clients in trauma counselling, often for the first time, exceed their capacity to automatically categorize, view and process the package of images, emotions and cognitions encysted within the traumatic experience. They have not developed cognitive or emotional literacy. After all, it is because the client's information-processing capacity was overwhelmed in the first place that he is now traumatized. However, that does not mean that, in the safety of a counselling environment and with the help of a counsellor, he is not now able to process the experience virtually on his own. It is for the counsellor to judge when further directive questions or guidance is needed. In keeping with the model used with TIR, such interventions should be kept to the **minimum necessary to help the client process the experience and no more**.

The repetitive nature of TIR enables the client to gradually dismantle whatever mental defences remain and access or recover the still sensitized, unviewed, or unprocessed material. When sufficient material is not being contacted by the client to produce a resolution, it is often because he needs direction of what to look at rather than because of 'resistance' to looking at the material. For example, the client might go through the incident several times, describing the visual images and actions in detail but not mentioning what he felt or thought during the trauma. In this case, the client may need to be asked to go through the incident again, recalling and describing what he was feeling at each stage and then what he was thinking at each stage. The client may go through the incident contacting its emotional content, but just replaying this in successive passes. In this case, the client may need to be asked to go through the incident again, paying attention to what he saw, then what he did, and then what he was thinking at the time.

However, counsellors should beware of **insisting** that a client should demonstrate a recovery of all the material theoretically contained within the trauma. The emotional content might already have been discharged in a debriefing, either formal or informal. It might not be significant compared with the cognitive content. Conversely, it may be that the client has already, by himself or with others, processed the cognitive content but not confronted the emotional content and needs directions and help to do so. Traumatic incidents are likely to have been extensively thought about and may be spoken about before the client arrives in counselling. It is the counsellor's job to enable the client to access and process those features of the incident that remain uncontacted and expressed when the client does not automatically do so. However, the counsellor must not intervene in an effort to 'speed things up'. As long as the session is progressing, e.g. the material is changing, the counsellor should not intervene.

Accessing involves directing the client when needed to qualia recorded at the time of the trauma and uninspected. Processing involves the client's conscious inspection of that qualia and determination of its meaning, consequences, associations and connections as needed to afford integration with earlier experience and his world view.

As stated earlier, accessing or recovering the detailed content of the trauma is accomplished by having the client repeatedly going through and recounting the incident. Access (as well as processing) can be aided with the use of prompting questions which re-orient the client to the incident. The work by Geiselman, Fisher, MacKinnon and Holland (1985) showed that in 'cognitive interviews' up to 30 per cent more information could be accurately recalled using four basic principles:

1. Asking the person to think back to immediately preceding events, his actions and his mood.
2. Having the person repeat every detail, however trivial.
3. Having the person describe events in different orders – both forwards and backwards.*
4. Asking the person to describe the event from different viewpoints.

Our experience has been that in TIR procedure, numbers 3 and 4 above have not proved necessary (but could be used if needed). However, both

---

* It should be noted that Whitten and Leonard (1981) showed that a backward-ordered search in memory was more effective than a forward-ordered or random search. The search for incidents in TIR is always conducted from the present backwards and time lines are constructed in the same way.

accessing and processing more often require the use of additional questions in line with 1 and 2 above.

The repeated reviewing and recounting of the incident in TIR facilitates an unburdening of its encapsulated mental energy or 'charge'. Although not the subject of research, experience suggests that there is a scale of difficulty in recalling the qualia contained within a traumatic memory. Most clients find it easy to recall the event, followed by how they felt, followed by what they thought. In recovering the incident, it seems best first to address and discharge the visual images and, second, the emotional content, at which point the cognitive content should be available. Ideally this happens automatically, but where it does not, prompter questions are used.

As Ellis (1958) has said, emotion and thinking are not easily separated being so interrelated as to operate in a circular cause and effect relationship. However, for the purposes of enabling clients to identify, categorize and make sense of the qualia encysted in the trauma, we need to differentiate in language at least. The following is a list of the main categories of qualia which are thought to have a potentially significant role in keeping a traumatic memory sensitized:

- Sensory information contained in the incident: including visual images of the incident itself, sounds in the incident (prominent and background), smells in the incident.
- Visual images imagined during the incident.
- Visual images of past experiences triggered during the incident.
- Physiological sensations or pains experienced in the incident.
- Focus of attention during the incident, any conflict of focus, what was he aware of happening that he was unable to pay attention to at the time.
- Intentions throughout the incident (conflicting, unfulfilled, suppressed).
- Actions taken during the incident, including any that were regretted and why, plus any he wanted to take and couldn't or didn't.
- Emotional state during the incident, change of state, emotional reactions.
- Strategies, either automatically or consciously deployed, to cope with the incident, the consequences of these strategies, what would have been preferred, what would have been worse.
- Cognitions: thoughts, assumptions, decisions, beliefs, expectations, ideas and conclusions made during the incident – or since the incident.
- Mysteries – information not available to him at the time or at all (see Chapter 2).
- People or things that should have been present at the time but were not. People and things that were present at the time but should not

have been. Events that should have taken place but didn't. Events that took place but should not have. In a word – incongruities.

- Practical questions arising out of the incident. (See Chapter 2. Practical and existential questions fall under the heading of 'unfinished business' and would be explored as needed.)
- Existential questions arising out of the incident.
- Anything the person wanted to communicate but did not or could not during or after the incident.
- Anything the person may have found out about himself (or concluded about himself) as a result of the incident (positive or negative).

As needed, the counsellor forms his own questions to enable the client to access material that so far has not been addressed and is not forthcoming. For example, 'You said you were feeling apprehensive up until the car actually crashed, but not what you felt then and afterwards. Please describe your feelings at the time.' Another example: 'Did you imagine or form any expectations of what was going to happen after the car went out of control?'

Here are some further examples:

- 'How did you react when told that your passenger was injured?'
- 'You mentioned that you "prayed and nothing happened". What were you feeling at the time?'
- 'Did you conclude anything from that experience?'
- 'Did this experience raise questions for you?'
- 'What were your immediate thoughts at the time?'
- 'When you shouted at the policeman, was that just an automatic response or was there a specific objective to that action?'
- 'You didn't mention any expression of emotion when your mother arrived. Was there any?'
- 'Did you try to hide your feelings?'
- 'Was there anything you wanted to say at the time and didn't?'
- 'Was there anything you wanted to do at the time and didn't?'
- 'Were you aware of anything else going on around you while you were trying to stop the bleeding?'

When using such questions, the counsellor should avoid getting into a discussion of that feature of the incident. The idea is to recover that feature and incorporate it into the narrative where it can be integrated with the information already addressed. Focusing on interesting parts of the incident before the whole has been reviewed and reduced can lead to the client settling on a partial insight and/or avoiding some other uncomfortable feature of the event, and premature closure could result. Again, the rule of thumb is if the incident is changing (e.g. either the content, focus, emotional content, or cognitive content) each time it is viewed, there is no need for any additional questions. It is only when the movement stops that prompting is needed.

Here is another example. John was working on an incident in which he was mugged in the street. He has reviewed the incident four times with little change and his focus was on the details of the incident without any emotional or cognitive content. The following is an excerpt from the session:

Please tell me what happened.

I was walking down Jump Road. I heard footsteps behind me. A man grabbed me and said 'Give me your money or I will kill you'. I felt a gun in my back. I gave the man all my money. The man let go of me and ran off. (No change at all from previous reviews – all said in a conversational tone.)

OK. What were you thinking at the time?

Nothing really.

Fine. Was there anything you believed was going to happen at the time of the incident?

Yes. I was sure I was going to be killed. I could feel the gun and I was positive that no matter what I did I was going to die. (John is shaking now.) *I was terrified* (John is crying) *and I felt like a coward.*

OK. Please go back to the beginning of the incident.

OK.

Good. Move through the incident again until you reach the end.

OK.

Good. Please tell me what happened.

I was walking down Jump Road. I was late and was hurrying. It was very dark out and I was feeling a bit insecure. I heard footsteps behind me and I wondered what they were. I remembered that a friend had been attacked on this road the week before, so I started walking faster . . . (John continued and eventually came to an end point.)

(End of excerpt.)

The Period Just Before and Just After the Incident

In many cases, one or more of the questions described earlier in this chapter will get the session moving again, and the counsellor will not need to ask any further questions or do anything else as the session will proceed to an end point. However, there are occasions where it is useful to examine the period just before the incident or just after the incident. For example, sometimes a client will not include the trip to hospital just following the actual road traffic accident or attack as part of the same incident. In other cases, the way people treated someone just after an incident can have more impact than the incident itself (such as when someone's boss was rude or dismissive or a family member was unsupportive). Sometimes, although the counsellor has spent time with the client to establish what happened just before the impact of the incident, not enough of this period will be examined during the session. This can be particularly significant for the client in situations in which surprise was a central factor – for example, when the person was on her way to a pleasant event and was then in a bad road traffic accident, or in the case of a client having had a prior intuition or precognition that something was going to occur.

In these situations, the counsellor can request the client to go to the period just before the incident occurred, or just after the incident occurred, and ask the following questions:

1. Where were you?
2. What were you doing?
3. Who was with you?
4. What were they doing?
5. What were your expectations at the time?

Also, the counsellor can ask any of the additional questions mentioned in this chapter. Once the counsellor has done this, he should go back to the regular TIR method until an end point is achieved.

Often what is presented as the trauma turns out to be less important or significant than preceding or following events, and requires special attention (as detailed above). For example, a client's wartime experience included a 24-hour waiting period during which his cognitive and emotional reactions proved to be much more significant than being shot and wounded afterwards. Counsellors need to be aware that their own perception of a traumatic event may differ considerably from the client's perception. Counsellors should be prepared to target TIR procedure on either preceding events or events following 'the trauma'.

In the next chapter, we discuss what the counsellor can do when the session does not go smoothly as planned.

9

WHEN THINGS DON'T GO AS PLANNED

The first section of the book (Chapters 1 to 4) set the scene for the use of TIR and related techniques. We gave the context for the use of these techniques with trauma and with Post-Traumatic Stress Disorder. We covered the start of the counselling relationship, including a detailed look at the assessment phase of our treatment. In the second section (Chapters 5 to 8) we focused on Unblocking and TIR and covered the basic techniques with detailed instructions and examples for their use. In this, the final section of the book, we examine more complex cases where things may not go as planned, and cover the end of the counselling.

Ideally, a TIR or Unblocking session will proceed smoothly as described. The client will choose the area he wants to examine, the counsellor will conduct the session as per the instructions, the client will reach an end point, both client and counsellor will leave the session feeling good about the work they have done, and the area examined will remain resolved to the degree stated – no longer such a problem to the client. This seems to happen most of the time.

There will of course be times – however well intentioned the client and the counsellor – when things do not proceed smoothly. In some of these situations, advanced techniques are needed to facilitate the client's progress. As far as TIR is concerned, some of these techniques can be learned in further books and workshops. Often if supervision is sought from a counsellor who has more experience working in this way, the supervisor can help by going over the particular situation and making suggestions. In some of these situations, TIR was not the appropriate choice for that particular client at that particular time. In these situations, referral to a supervisor can verify this and another treatment method suggested. In some situations the session does not proceed smoothly because of an error on the part of the counsellor. In this chapter, the most common errors and ways of correcting them are covered.

TIR involves helping a client to compartmentalize his experience and examine it piece by piece. This is a very important facet of TIR, making it possible for the client to examine his experience in manageable chunks. Clients have often remarked that their entire lives are traumatic and that they find it difficult to separate where one incident ends and the next one begins. During the assessment phase, the history-taking and time line help the client to see these divisions more clearly. This usually is a relief to the client – as his experience no longer resembles a tangle of moss but begins to look more like a spider's web. The structure in TIR serves the same function. The idea of finishing a piece of work – recognizing when something is resolved – is central to this structure. If the counsellor does not recognize the end point and continues the session, the client will oblige – usually by finding a related area to examine. This can result in the client *over*-analysing an experience and getting bogged down in the significance of the experience, rather than having appreciated its essence and moving on. Incidents can be over-examined as well as under-examined.

If a cake is left in the oven too long, it burns and becomes inedible. If a session goes on for too long, it can become confusing, the client can become exhausted and no resolution will be reached. The counsellor should suspect that an end point has been missed when he sees any of the following:

1. At some point during the session, the counsellor saw most of the indicators that signal an end point (for example: the area was much lighter, the client reported that he was feeling better, the client's attention moved to the external environment).
2. Following this, the client began to look worse and not one of the indicators of an end point was present.
3. When the counsellor checked for an earlier connected incident, there was none but there continued to be no change on the present incident.

If the counsellor notices these points, then to confirm that he has missed the end point, he asks the client 'Were you feeling better about this incident at some point during this session?' or 'Was there a point during this session at which this felt resolved?'. If the counsellor has missed the end point, the client will look visibly relieved and respond that there was, and will usually tell the counsellor when that was and may even describe what he concluded at that point during the session. At that point, the counsellor could apologize for missing the end point. For example, he says 'I'm sorry. We should have ended the session at that point.' If the client does not demonstrate the indicators of the end point once the counsellor has established that an end point was missed, then, prior to ending the session, he encourages the client to talk about the end point that was missed; for example, 'What were you feeling at that point in the session?', 'What were you thinking at that point in the session?'. The counsellor ends the session as soon as the client is looking well and demonstrating that an end point has been reached. This is not usually a long process and it is important that the counsellor does not spend too long on it. The point of the process is to allow the client to acknowledge the point of resolution. The session should then be ended. The important issue here is that, at any point in 'processing' an incident, the client may come to a realization that resolves it for her. Such a point can easily be missed by the counsellor (particularly if she has her own ideas about what 'resolution' consists of).

A 'point of resolution' is a *process* phenomenon. It may not be the end of the issue for all time (something a counsellor might want to achieve) but is a point that the client feels has resolved that particular issue at that time and, if ignored, would result in grinding over and over something in which the client has now no interest.

THE MOST COMMON ERRORS IN TIR

The following are the most common errors made by counsellors who have just started using TIR. Along with a description of the error is a description of how to correct the error. Many counsellors find they are able to recognize these errors when reviewing their session notes and can correct the error in the same session or in the next session. If the counsellor is not sure what has happened, a supervisor will usually be able to recognize these errors from a session tape or transcript. In some situations it may be necessary for the counsellor to get more information from the client before the error can be identified and then corrected. In other cases, more than one thing is going wrong and all the difficulties will need to be corrected to bring the issue to resolution.

Stopping the Session Too Early

This is one of the most common errors we see with counsellors who have just learned to use TIR. Counsellors become quite concerned about going on too long and will end a session before an end point has been reached. Often the counsellor becomes mired in the content of the session and loses the thread of the process. In TIR the client and his process is more important than the content of the session. We examine content when we are looking for a cognitive shift because, by definition, we must examine the content of the cognitive elements of the session in order to decide if there has been a shift. However, there are many cognitive shifts during the average TIR session. A cognitive shift that signifies that the end point is approaching is usually a major shift and a shift in an adaptive direction.

For example, the following session excerpt illustrates a variety of shifts in cognition that occurred during a TIR session and the shift at the point of resolution.

This was one of Mary's sessions in which she examined two incidents where her father humiliated her in front of the family when she was 12 years old. The incidents involved her father sitting in a chair reading pornographic novels (silently) and having Mary stand in front of him so he could look at her. She was told to stand still and was aware that he was aroused and was horrified by it.

After she had been through the incident twice she said the following:

He keeps threatening to send me away. I'd do anything not to be sent away to a hospital which is where he says he'll send me. (Mary sighs.) *The goal posts keep changing with him – this is why I always feel on edge – then and now.*

That was the first cognitive shift where Mary made a connection between that incident, the theme of the incident and present-day symptoms. However, she was still extremely upset and crying, and the incident did not feel resolved. This is an example of a shift during the session. The other indications of an end point are not present, so the session continues. After a few more times through the incident Mary says the following:

He never did send me away. (Mary laughs.) *I suppose it is very hard to replace slaves.* (Mary laughs; she is sitting more relaxed in the chair, the colour has returned to her face.) *Basically during that time period, I did the best I could. I was damned if I did and damned if I didn't. Because of that I grew up with no idea what I wanted and the idea that in order to be safe I had to be able to read minds. I learned to do whatever it takes – and have always done that – stayed in situations much longer than I needed to – compromised where I shouldn't have – endangered myself – because I didn't feel I could do anything differently – I was damned either way. The positive side was determination – do whatever it takes to succeed. I don't have to be that way any more. I don't have to read minds – I can ask!* (Mary is smiling and making eye contact with the counsellor.) *That feel's great.*

At this point, the counsellor ended the session. The cognitive shift included an understanding of her decisions and cognitive process at the time of the incident, how it continued to affect her adult life and a decision to change. Not all cognitive shifts leading to end points will look like this. Some are much more subtle. The counsellor becomes more confident as she gets to know her client and how her client processes and expresses material.

There are times where a session is ended prior to an end point. As mentioned previously, this occurs when the session has gone on for a long time (defined as longer than 1 hour and 45 minutes) and an end point is unlikely to be reached before the client tires (e.g. within three to four hours) or where there is too much connected and highly charged material to finish in one session of reasonable length (not longer than four hours in session). In these situations, the counsellor ends the session at a place where the incident has levelled out – it is less charged than when the client entered the session and is desensitized. Both the client and the counsellor are usually aware that the incident or group of incidents will have to be revisited in the next session. In our experience, this is more of an exception than a rule. Counsellors using TIR must remember not to end a session for their convenience, but according to the client's process. An average TIR session lasts 90 minutes.

If a counsellor has ended a session before an end point, sometimes the client will continue to talk about the incident after session (and before he leaves the room). If this happens, the counsellor should continue where they left off in the next TIR session. Often the counsellor is not aware that he has ended the session too early until he examines his session notes or speaks with a supervisor. If he notices this, he should revisit the incident in the next session. Sometimes when talking with the client at the beginning of a following session to clear up anything that is currently attracting the client's attention, the counsellor discovers that he ended the previous session too soon. If the client brings up the previous session and is not speaking about the positive new things he has realized since that session, then the counsellor should revisit the incident. If the counsellor is concerned he may have ended the previous session too early, he can ask the client how he has felt about the incident(s) they worked on during that session. If the client becomes upset, or talks about spending time thinking about the incidents (in anything other than a positive way), then the counsellor should revisit the incident(s).

Some clients tend to do a lot of processing between sessions. Usually they see this as positive – their thoughts about the incident(s) are not perceived as intrusive but rather as continuing to fit things into place and to make sense of things. We find that as we work with a client, we become familiar with his style and this makes it easier to discriminate between further processing and unfinished material. The rule of thumb is, if there is a negative or intrusive element to the client's thinking about the incident outside of session, then the incident or group of incidents should be revisited.

Missing the End Point

We examined this at the beginning of the chapter. The counsellor must beware of revisiting incidents that are resolved for the client. If the client has no interest in examining an incident or says that it feels fine, the counsellor must take this seriously, respect the client and not insist on revisiting the incident. Below is an example from an actual client:

(The subject of the TIR session was a rape when Jane was 18 years old. There was considerable emotion for the first six times through the incident and considerable cognitive change. The excerpt begins on the seventh time through the incident. As in previous transcripts, Jane's material is in *italics* and the counsellor's material or observations are in regular print.)

. . . I just realized that this is past now. I cannot forgive him but it is in the past. (Tone of voice is calm and definite; colour has returned to the face.)

OK. Please go back to the start of the incident.

Yes.

Move through the incident again step by step silently.

OK.

Please tell me what happened.

I'm finding this boring – the incident is still the same. Nothing happened this time.

OK. Let's go over the incident again. The beginning was when you were in the room.

OK.

Go through the incident step by step silently.

OK. (Looks annoyed; is fidgeting.)

Please tell me what happened.

Nothing. I'm bored with this. I'm not sure what difference it makes. I won't forgive him but it is not a problem.

Was there a point while we've been doing this where you felt better about this incident?

Yes. (Brightens up.) *When I realized it was in the past.*

OK. Sorry about that. We should have ended there.

That's OK. (Brighter but not as relaxed as previously.)

Tell me a bit about what you realized at that point.

Well, I won't forgive him – which is fine. But the incident is over now and I can get on with my life. I feel peaceful about it.

Good. We'll end the session here.

Fine. Thanks.

(End of excerpt.)

Missing an Earlier Connection

As discussed earlier, TIR is built on the idea that traumatic events are often connected to each other in a variety of ways and that the best way of resolving a particular event may involve examining that event as well as those connected events that occurred earlier in time in the same session. If an incident has been examined on its own in a session and the incident continues to trouble the client, it is possible that an earlier connection has been missed. Sometimes the client will spontaneously bring up the earlier incident in the following session. For example, Joe worked on a road traffic accident he experienced in 1990 in one session. A full end point was not reached during the session but Joe felt considerably better about the accident and the session was ended after two and a half hours. In the week following the session, Joe had nightmares about a road traffic accident he experienced in 1982. When he attended his next session, he told the counsellor about these nightmares. The counsellor used TIR on the accident in 1982 and a full end point was reached.

Other times, the client will be unaware that an earlier connection has been missed. This is particularly common when the incidents do not appear to be obviously connected (as two road traffic accidents, or two fights, or two incidents of abuse might be) but are connected by themes or by sensory stimuli. Sometimes the earlier connection will surface during the first TIR session, but the client may dismiss this because he thinks it is irrelevant. Again, it is important to remind a client to tell you whatever comes to mind, even if it seems irrelevant, as experience tells us that if it comes to mind, there is usually a connection (which often becomes obvious only by the time the client has reached an end point).

One clue that an earlier connection may have been missed is the incident continuing to trouble the client following the TIR session. The counsellor can check this in the next TIR session by having the client review the incident again until there is no further change (often only a couple of times) and then asking the client if there is an earlier connected incident and reminding the client to tell him whatever comes to mind. Usually the client will mention an earlier incident at this point and TIR can be continued until an end point is reached.

Sometimes this possibility is picked up in supervision when a session has not ended well – a point of resolution was not reached. The supervisor will sometimes suggest that the counsellor check with the client to make sure no earlier connection was missed. The counsellor must keep in mind that, in many cases, incidents are not connected in obvious and logical ways. In addition, clients will often volunteer earlier incidents that were not on their original trauma lists or do not appear to be traumatic. Remember that as the awareness threshold lowers, the client has access to more material.

In thematic TIR, there are almost always a number of earlier connected incidents. By definition, if one is looking at a theme, there are a number of different instances in which that theme was present. This is why, in thematic work, the counsellor looks for earlier connections much more quickly than when doing TIR with a presenting incident. If a client has only examined one or two incidents when in a thematic TIR session, it is likely that earlier connections have not been examined. In this case, in the next session, the counsellor just starts TIR with the theme again. If there are no earlier connections, the client will usually have no interest in the theme and no further action is needed.

The Client's Attention was Distracted by Something Else

Sometimes sessions go poorly because the client's attention was actually on some recent event or problem in his environment when the session began. This is more likely to happen if the counsellor forgets to ask the client about his current situation at the beginning of the session. If the counsellor is unsure of what is going wrong during a session, he can ask the client 'Is there anything your attention is on at the moment?' or 'Has something crossed your mind that you haven't mentioned?', and if this is the problem, the client will often tell him at that point. Once the counsellor has discovered what the distraction is, he must do something to deal with it before proceeding with the TIR session. Sometimes this involves a considerable amount of work and the TIR session must be abandoned, at other times it merely causes a short delay before the session can be resumed. For example, if the client had a telephone call to make at 3 p.m. and he is aware that considerable time has passed, he may have his attention on the telephone call. If the counsellor finds this to be the case, he can tell the client the time and take a session break to enable the client to make the telephone call. The counsellor can then resume the session. However, if the client had a large row with his wife just prior to session and they are trying to do TIR on a road traffic accident, it may be necessary for the counsellor to abandon the TIR session in favour of working with the client on the row and/or his relationship with his wife.

The rule of thumb is that you can only work on what the client has his attention on. You cannot ask the client to split his attention and expect to get good results with TIR. TIR takes considerable mental energy and attention. It would also go against the principle of working on one area at a time. If the counsellor explores how the client is and anything his attention is on prior to starting TIR, this should not happen.

The Client is Withholding Information from the Counsellor

Sometimes the client will dismiss what comes to mind as irrelevant and feel that it is not necessary to mention it to the counsellor during the session. This can get in the way of the progress of the session, particularly if the client's attention is on the information he is not disclosing to the counsellor. Sometimes the client chooses not to disclose something to the counsellor because he is concerned about how the counsellor will react, or because he feels unable to say the words out loud. In both of these cases, the session could grind to a halt. This is primarily because the client is focused on what he is not saying rather than on viewing the traumatic material. The counsellor can encourage the client to tell him what he is withholding by asking any of the following questions:

- 'Is there anything that has crossed your mind that you have not mentioned?'
- 'Has something occurred to you that you haven't mentioned?'
- 'Is there something your attention has been fixed upon?'
- 'Has something come to mind that you found it difficult to tell me?'

(Note: These are examples, the counsellor can construct his own questions. It is important that the questions are not felt to be 'punitive' by the client, e.g., 'Are you lying to me?' would not be a good question.)

If it turns out that there is something the client does not feel he can disclose, then it may be necessary for the counsellor to work on safety issues with the client before the TIR session can continue. If necessary, this could involve having the client write down the material he feels he cannot say. If this feels too difficult for the client, then the counsellor can explore the client's fears and concerns and provide reassurance where necessary. If this is not working, a supervisor can provide other techniques designed to help the client become more comfortable in his communication with the counsellor. This is a rare occurrence. Adequate time should have been spent in history-taking to have provided for a good therapeutic alliance.

Again, what is important is the way the process is affected by the client withholding material. It is the fact that the client's attention becomes split – part on what he is withholding and part on the TIR material that causes the problem. The content is often completely unconnected to the TIR material the client is reviewing. For example, one client found the counsellor very attractive. In the middle of a TIR session, this thought ran through his mind. He was too embarrassed to tell the counsellor. His attention then switched from the incident he was reviewing to the counsellor and his thoughts about the counsellor. The session ground to a halt. The counsellor had noticed that his attention had appeared to wander and asked the client, 'Is there something that has crossed your mind that you haven't mentioned to me?' At this point the client blushed (an indication that confirmed the counsellor was correct in thinking that there was something the client was not saying). After a pause, the client finally said that he thought he found her very attractive. The counsellor responded by acknowledging the client and then asked the client to return to the incident. The client was relieved that the counsellor had not been offended; he was able to return his attention to the incident he was examining and the session proceeded.

In the previous example, all that was needed was for the comment to be made and the session could then continue. In other cases, as in the example of the telephone call, some action will have to be taken on the part of the counsellor before the session can be resumed. In some cases, the client withholds the fact that he is bored with the incident. In this case, it is particularly important for the counsellor to have this information as it influences what the counsellor does next. As mentioned earlier, boredom can have many meanings in a session – including that an end point has been missed. Counsellors should investigate non-verbal communication when they feel or observe that the client is not engaged in the incident. When the client *is* engaged, then the counsellor should do nothing.

Remember that the client needs to feel safe enough in his relationship with the counsellor to tell the counsellor whatever crosses his mind. If the counsellor has refrained from judging the client (even in her non-verbal reactions to the client) and refrained from interpreting for the client, then the client is more likely to feel safe enough.

Observation is a counsellor's best tool for noticing when a client is withholding something in a session. If all of a counsellor's attention is focused on the client, then he is more likely to observe changes that indicate that the client's attention has shifted – which indicates that something may have occurred to the client that he has not yet expressed. Keep in mind that clients often withhold information unintentionally – because they feel it is irrelevant, or because they have not yet fully processed the information and so haven't yet expressed it. TIR sessions should not feel like interrogations. Space for the client to process material should be given, and questions should be asked only when there has been an obvious shift in attention or when the client appears to be adrift.

BAND AIDS (PLASTERS)

Band aids are techniques that are used to help close a session down when a full end point has not been reached but there is a reason that the session must be ended. The following are reasons for ending a session short of a full end point:

1. The client is very tired.
2. You have run short of time – either because the client has another appointment, or you have another appointment. (Note: This should be avoided if at all possible. It is not good practice to schedule sessions less than two hours apart or to end sessions based on next appointments.)
3. The session is not going well and supervision is needed to figure out how to remedy it.
4. The client was not in shape for session to begin with, but this was not discovered until the middle of the session (e.g. the client has not eaten, is hung over, has a bad headache that began prior to the session).

The purpose of a 'band aid' is to help the client bring his attention back into the present and focus on the external environment. Anything that achieves this goal can be used as a band aid. We recommend a variety of ways of achieving this goal in this section, but if the reader has a preferred method already, then that could be used.

Educating the Client on Band Aids

In our experience, it is better to educate the client about the use of band aids in general so that there is no mystery. Again, this empowers the client, enabling him to cooperate in the exercise rather than disempowering him so that he feels the counsellor is 'doing something to' him.

Educating the client on band aids does not have to be an extensive activity. It can be as simple as telling the client that, from time to time, he might be asked to focus on pleasant experiences or to focus on objects in the immediate physical environment, and that this serves the purpose of helping him to be more grounded in the present before a session is ended and he has to go back out into the world. Even when sessions go well, clients can be lost somewhere in their mental environments and appear somewhat 'spacey' or 'out of it' at the end of a session. It is a good idea to help the client reorient to the present and the environment – particularly if he has to get in a car and drive home.

Recalling Pleasant Experiences

One way of helping a client to close down and ground if he is still in a negative part of the incident is to have him recall pleasant life experiences. If he is still in a negative part of his mental environment, the object is to have the client move from the past to recent pleasant experiences. The counsellor is asking the client to look at a mental photograph rather than a video or movie. It is best to keep this quick – to keep the client from looking at a movie – because pleasant experiences can often be surrounded by unpleasant ones. Life is a continuum with pleasant and unpleasant experiences all mixed together and you do not want the client to trigger another unpleasant or traumatic memory while you are trying to close a session down.

French and Gerbode provide a prepared list of instructions in *The Traumatic Incident Reduction Workshop* (1995) which is revised and reprinted with permission below. This list can be quite effective with many clients, particularly if the material they have been examining in session is related to negative experiences with other people. However, there are some liabilities to using this list. If a client has always had troubled relationships with others then he might find this list more upsetting than uplifting. If the counsellor has any doubt that this will work well, then he is better off creating a less threatening list – one that has nothing to do with relationships with other human beings.

Remembering Pleasant Experiences

You can use this list of instructions to close down a session if you are unable to bring the session to an end point. Use the list before ending the session for a consultation with a supervisor. Take it to a point where the client feels better and has his attention in the present. This may only take one question. Once the client has reoriented his attention, then that is an end point. On this list you are asking for a brief photograph or snapshot rather than the entire story. If necessary, you can go through the list more than once. Remember that an end point on this list is not the same as reaching the end point for the incident you were working on which resulted in your using this list. You must still finish that action in a later session. Ask the client to remember:

1. A time when you confided in someone.
2. A time when you felt very close to someone.
3. A time when you were communicating well with someone.
4. A time when someone confided in you.
5. A time when someone was communicating well with you.
6. A time when someone really liked you.
7. A time when you really liked someone.
8. A time when the world seemed very vivid to you.
9. A time when you were in good control of a situation.
10. A time when someone really understood you.
11. A time when you really understood someone.
12. A recent time when you shared someone's world.
13. A recent time when someone shared your world.
14. A recent time when you really liked someone.
15. A recent time when someone was really fond of you.
16. A recent time when you felt close to someone.
17. A recent time when you felt a strong sense of reality.
18. A recent time when you understood someone.
19. A recent time when someone really understood you.
20. A recent time when you were in good control of things.

Sometimes we use only one instruction, repeatedly to accomplish the same goal – bringing the client back into the present and into a more pleasant state. For example: 'Remember a time when you enjoyed yourself' or 'Remember a time when you felt happy and peaceful' or 'Remember a time when you helped someone.'

To create an individual list, choose non-threatening material for that client. For example, if the client enjoys animals and has not suffered from the bereavement of a pet, you could ask the client to remember pleasant experiences with animals. For example:

1. A recent time when you stroked a dog.
2. A recent time when you played with a rabbit.
3. A recent time when you saw a beautiful bird.
4. A recent time when you heard birds singing.

We have often used sensory-based lists – including enjoyed foods, enjoyed scents, enjoyed textures, enjoyed sights and enjoyed sounds. For example:

1. A recent time when you saw a lovely sunset.
2. A recent time when you smelled a flower.
3. A recent time when you tasted rich chocolate.
4. A recent time when you ate your favourite dessert.

Again, it is important to move quickly through this list of instructions. You do not want the client to focus for too long on any one incident. Any list you create should ask for recent experiences towards the end, as the idea is to bring the client back into the present. The list should not be very long.

If a counsellor prefers to use a conversational method to examine pleasant experiences, this will work just as well. Again, the counsellor should not spend too long on any one subject. For example, the excerpt below is taken from a session with Mary, which went very well and an end point was reached, but she was very light-headed when the session finished and not in condition to leave the office to make her way home. Again, the counsellor's material is in regular print and Mary's material is in *italics*.

What do you feel like for dinner this evening when you get home?

I really feel like a take-away meal – and then a nice pudding.

What kind of take-away do you feel like most?

I really enjoy Chinese.

When was the last time you had a Chinese take-away?

It was about six months ago. I had aromatic crispy duck. (Mary is smiling, making eye contact with the counsellor.)

I find that a delicious dish. What other Chinese food do you enjoy?

I like most Chinese food. I also like Indian. (At this point Mary is looking much more in the present and the counsellor winds the conversation down.)

Indian is nice too. So which are you going to have tonight?

Chinese. I can't wait.

OK. Which train are you catching?

(Looks at watch.) *I best leave now or I'll miss it.*

(End of excerpt.)

Grounding Techniques: Making the Client More Aware of His Surroundings

Another band aid is grounding techniques. These are designed to help the client reconnect with his present external environment. They usually work quite quickly. They can be used to close down an incomplete session, at the end of a heavy session in which an end point has been reached, and during a TIR session if the client experiences some negative phenomena such as dissociation or headaches or other physical sensations and these are not disappearing by completing the procedure (which is what usually happens).

Use at the End of a Session

If the session has gone well and an end point has been reached, it should only be necessary to use a few instructions before the client feels centred and grounded in the present and in his environment. If the session is incomplete or has not gone well, it may take longer before the client feels grounded in the present external environment. Below are some suggestions for the counsellor; however, the counsellor should feel free to compile his own to suit the client.

Grounding refers to helping the client move his attention to the external environment. Ideally when a session has been taken to an end point, then the client's attention has moved from his internal (mental) environment (introspected) to having attention on the external environment (extrospected).

Grounding in the Visual Environment

The counsellor should explain the purpose of this exercise to the client before he does it. We often tell clients that they may find this odd or strange, and that is fine. We remind clients to tell us whatever comes to mind when doing the exercise. Give each instruction, wait for the client's response, and then acknowledge the response before giving the next instruction. Ask the client to look at objects in the immediate physical environment. Make sure not to be overcomplicated. Have the client look at objects in all parts of the room, one by one, moving relatively quickly. An example of this at the end of a session might take the following form (this is an excerpt from an actual client; as previously, the counsellor's material is in regular print and the client's material is in *italics*):

(An end point was reached but the client is still feeling somewhat lightheaded and the session was quite intense.)

The next thing we are going to do is completely different. The purpose is to help you feel centred and grounded in the present and in the external environment – to take you from inside your head to being aware of things outside your head. Does that make sense to you?

You mean from thinking about my stuff to being aware of the world around me?

Yes. I'm going to ask you to look at various things in the room. I want you to tell me whatever comes to mind, including 'This is stupid!'. There is no hidden agenda here – we are just helping you to feel more grounded. OK?

OK. I'm already feeling a bit silly.

That's fine, most people do. Please look at that curtain.

OK.

Good. Now please look at that brass ornament.

OK. (Looking around the room, looking a bit better.)

OK. Please look at that cheese plant.

God. It's huge. How did you ever get it to grow like that? I never really noticed how large it was!

(The counsellor notices the client's attention is firmly on the external environment and decides to answer the question and end the exercise.) It seems to just grow and grow. It won't fit in the room soon.

(Laughing.) *It will take over the house.*

(Laughing.) Yes it will. How are you feeling now?

Better. Much more centred.

OK. We'll stop here.

(End of excerpt.)

The counsellor must be sure to make instructions specific enough to be followed without the client having to guess what the counsellor wants. For example, if there are two sets of curtains in a room, 'Please look at the curtains' would not be a good instruction.

This exercise can be done with any sensory modality or with mixed modalities. When closing down an incomplete session, tactile instructions often work most quickly. We have a small bowl full of objects of various textures that we keep in the counselling room for these occasions. We explain the exercise in the same fashion but emphasize it is a way to help the client feel better before he or she leaves the session. The bowl of objects includes a piece of fur, a piece of sandpaper, a smooth stone, a rugged stone and a piece of cloth. Any variety of objects can be used. We often draw attention to the temperature of an object, and also use tactile objects, asking the client to touch the fabric of the settee or touch the carpet.

The counsellor can draw attention to colour, tone of sounds, texture or temperature of objects. The counsellor could even devise something using a variety of scents or flavours. As long as it is quick and easy and encourages the client to bring his attention from his internal environment to the external environment. Please note that we would not use this in a situation where the external environment was unpleasant (for example, at the scene of an accident), but we have used this in crisis intervention situations.

This can also be done using a conversational approach, by starting a conversation with a client about a particular object in the room or something that can be seen out of a window. In order to do this, there must be something that could be of enough interest to sustain a conversation around it. For example, it would be hard to get the client engaged in discussing the carpet unless it is an antique rug and the client takes an interest in such things. We have pointed out a garden scene from outside a window and drawn the client's attention to buds on trees and flowers beginning to open. It may not be easy to move to a conversational method without it seeming awkward and strange to the client unless the counsellor has practised it. If the client thinks it is strange, acknowledge that it is and explain the purpose of the exercise. More often than not, simply offering the client a cup of tea and having one is sufficient to ground the client after counselling (providing that counsellor and client do not discuss issues relating the client's therapy when drinking the tea). The keynote here is that when clients have gone through an abnormal experience, followed by another (i.e. counselling if they have had no previous experience of it), then sending them straight home could create another sense of unreality and they may still 'be in their heads'. The use of a cup of tea should not be underestimated.

Use in a TIR Session

We occasionally have clients who dissociate so much during a TIR session that they appear to move away and may develop a headache in the middle of the session. This appears to occur because the client moves from being in contact with the incident and his feelings, thoughts, and sensations, to being dissociated from the incident, and again being in contact with the incident, in very quick succession. When this occurs, grounding techniques can be very useful in helping this phenomena to ease to enable the client to continue the session. These techniques will not usually work when a headache has developed prior to the session. They seem to work only in cases of dissociation.

In these situations, we explain to the client what we are going to do and the purpose, as above, and then use 5–20 instructions. Usually, if this is going to work, it will work within 20 instructions. If it has not worked at that point and the client's symptoms are quite intense, we will usually end the session. The following is an example from an actual session.

(The session was a TIR session on a rape. On the seventh time through the incident, the client reported that she had a headache As usual, the counsellor's material is in regular print and the client's is in *italics*.)

OK. When did the headache start?

Just a few moments ago, but it is very bad.

OK. Remember, during the education, we discussed that sometimes during a TIR session you might experience physical sensations that occurred during the incident?

Yes.

Good. I said that if you did, the best thing we could do is to continue the session because usually if it starts during the session, continuing will make it stop.

Yes. I remember.

OK. I'd like you to tell me when the headache changes, OK?

Fine. (The client reviewed the incident three more times with the headache getting worse and stated she could not go on much longer.)

OK. What I'd like us to do is an exercise that might help your headache. It is designed to help you centre yourself and be more grounded. It may seem strange but don't worry, most people find it a bit strange. Are you willing to try?

Yes. Fine.

OK. I'm going to have you notice various things about the external environment. Please tell me whatever comes to mind as usual. Please look at that picture of a tree.

OK.

Good. Please look at that picture of a flower.

OK.

OK. Please listen to the sound of the birds outside the window.

Yes. That's pretty.

Good. Feel the texture of this piece of fur.

That's really soft.

OK. Please look at the glass sculpture.

OK.

Fine. Please look at the fabric-covered kaleidoscope.

So that's what it is. I hadn't realized. Can I look inside?

Yes. (Gives the client the kaleidoscope.) Pay attention to the colours in the patterns.

Yes. This is lovely. Are the others kaleidoscopes?

Yes. (Gives the client another kaleidoscope.) Notice the patterns this time.

Yes. Very nice.

How is your headache?

Gone actually. (Smiles.)

OK. (Smiles.) Are you ready to finish the session?

Yes. Fine.

Good. Go back to the beginning of the incident.

(End of excerpt.)

If the client reports a headache that started gradually in the session, we may continue with the session asking the client to let us know if it changes, and if it is necessary to discontinue the session. Sometimes we will remind clients that physical sensations can be triggered during the TIR (usually those experienced at the time of the incident) and that they are likely to disappear through continuing the TIR (as the counsellor did in the above excerpt). Obviously, if the sensation does not disappear or it is interfering with the client's ability to continue the session, the session is ended. However, when the sensations are things felt at the time of the incident, it is better if the session can be completed (e.g. a point of resolution reached) as this usually resolves the sensations. It is worth mentioning this when the counsellor educates the client, and reminding the client of the education if it occurs during a session. This is one of the reasons it is so important to educate the client – he will usually be much more willing to continue the session if he understands what is happening and is aware that continuing is more likely to resolve the sensations than stopping.

A Note about Relaxation and Guided Visualization Techniques

These can be useful aids to calming a client and to re-establishing feelings of safety and security. However, they have the liability of taking the client to another internal place rather than grounding the client in the external environment. For some clients, this does not appear to matter and these techniques are useful ways of closing down a session. However, these techniques can make other clients feel light-headed or 'not quite there' – which is not the desired result. In addition, there are clients who suffer from relaxation-induced anxiety. These clients feel the full weight of their anxiety only when they relax and tend to react poorly to relaxation techniques as a result. For these reasons, we prefer to use the band aids detailed in this chapter rather than using relaxation techniques.

10

ENDING THE
COUNSELLING

In this chapter we cover issues around ending treatment. We include
excerpts from the final sessions with both clients whom we have followed
in this book, together with their comments about the therapeutic process,
and discuss their follow-up test results.

THE 'END POINT' OF TRAUMA COUNSELLING

Deciding when it is appropriate to end a TIR session is a process –
oriented decision – and so, too, is the decision to end the counselling
relationship. One of the most obvious symptoms of traumatization is that
a substantial portion of the person's attention is preoccupied with past,
unprocessed experiences. When these have been successfully addressed
then attention is free to return to the present and the future. This is
usually a major and quite unmistakable shift. Frequently clients will bring
issues relating to their present lives to sessions throughout the counselling programme. However, when the end of counselling is approaching
(on a process level), these issues begin to take precedence and the client
will often introduce issues relating to future plans and goals (or concerns
about a lack of future plans). On a process level, this indicates that the
client now has enough attention and intention available to consider issues
relating to the future – attention and intention that has been released from
his past, by virtue of resolving past traumatic material.

Some clients are quite aware of this process and tell the counsellor that
they are ready to end the counselling relationship. We often schedule a
session to discuss the ending of the relationship, to retest clients (when
we are using psychometric tests) and then one follow-up session for one
or two months after the final session date. We offer the clients the option
of cancelling this session should they feel it is unnecessary, but explain
that we like to give them, and us, the opportunity to review the work we

have done together once they have resumed their lives. The follow-up session acknowledges the importance of the counselling relationship and gives the client the opportunity to report back on his successes, raise new issues that have arisen, and codify the results of his counselling experience. It also allows the client to give us feedback as to what was useful and what was not useful. In some settings, we provide an anonymous satisfaction survey for clients to complete and return by post. The survey, the psychometric testing, and the follow-up interview all allow us to continually monitor our efficacy and to learn from our experiences with clients.

Some clients are not too aware of the process and are unsure about when the counselling relationship should come to an end. This is particularly the case with clients who think that the counsellor will decide when they are 'better' or not (this despite education from us on this subject). Some clients retain the expectation that the counsellor knows best. In these cases, when we notice the shift from past to present and future, we schedule a session in which we go over the original trauma list and ask the client to re-rate the SUDs levels for the items on the list. This activity usually clarifies if there is more work to do or if the conclusion that the counselling relationship was drawing to a close was correct. Clients will often remark on the list, making comments that indicate that they are just beginning to realize how much has changed. For example, one client, when examining her original list, said 'I don't even remember putting that accident on the list – it has been such a long time since I thought about it! And I rated it a 10 at the time. A lot has changed!' Conversely, another client stated that 'I know we looked at the road traffic accident but it is still bothering me', which indicated that more work needed to be done on this incident.

In some cases it is clear that work needs to be done on the client's future goals and plans, or that new skills need to be acquired before the client will feel comfortable ending the counselling relationship. For such cases, we developed and often use a related structured method of working that focuses on goals and problem solving. We call this method 'Schema Programmes', which will be the subject of a future book.* When further work is necessary, we plan this work and discuss it with the client – educating the client as necessary. Once the work is completed, we plan the final sessions in the same way as we do when no further work has been necessary.

---

* We (and others) teach this method in a series of workshops and there are workshop manuals already published. For more information, contact the authors.

In some cases, a client has come for trauma counselling, and other long-term issues are raised during the counselling that are not fully addressed in the course of the counselling. In these cases, we may (with the client's agreement and providing it is within our expertise) choose to continue to work with the client on a longer term basis using different methods of working, or using other related methods of working. In these situations, we will always have at least one re-evaluation session with the client in order to determine what issues need addressing and to discuss how we might address these issues. In some circumstances, we will refer a client to another practitioner at this stage. For example, one client had long-term personality issues that did not prevent her from engaging in TIR and trauma work. Once the trauma work was complete, she identified the issues she felt needed to be addressed. She felt that she needed to work actively on her relationships with others and learn new skills for these relationships. Her relationships had been examined in the trauma counselling and considerable change had occurred as a result. However, she felt that there were some long patterns of behaviour and reaction that were not being addressed. The counsellor agreed and referred her for group therapy as the counsellor felt this was the most appropriate treatment modality to address these particular issues. In another case, the client still had some anxiety around using public transport. In this case it was appropriate to use *in vivo* exposure (literally 'in life' exposure) and the counsellor, who was experienced in this type of work, developed an *in vivo* programme to address this residual anxiety.

As we are involved in research, we collect psychometric testing data on our research clients at six months, one year and two years following completion of treatment. We advocate doing this with private clients as well, as it allows the counsellor to monitor efficacy. When we are able to, we also collect testing data from our private clients at regular intervals.

Some clients choose to leave counselling having only partially addressed the issues they brought into the counselling. Unless we believe the client is in imminent danger (e.g. he is having suicidal or homicidal thoughts or feelings), we respect the client's decision. Because we stress the distinction between the client as a whole person and his 'baggage' (the material in his mental environment that he has brought to counselling), we usually find that clients are willing to return for further counselling at a future date without feeling as though either they or we have failed. In addition, they tend not to express embarrassment at requesting further work as they are aware that we do not see this as unusual or as a sign that the original work was not useful or complete in and of itself.

RESULTS FROM MARY

Mary was quite aware of her own process through the trauma counselling. After 15.5 hours of counselling, the counsellor presented her with her trauma list to choose the next incident to work on and Mary stated, 'There is nothing here that bothers me anymore.' The rest of the session was spent discussing the changes that had occurred since Mary began the counselling and at the end a follow-up testing session was arranged. Below is an excerpt from this final session.

It is amazing looking at this list because, when I first looked at the list, I would become upset immediately – just by looking at it. Now, nothing jumps off the page, nothing on this list bothers me. It is all in the past and my attention is on the future. (Mary is laughing, relaxed posture, eye contact is good.)

That's good news. I am really pleased for you. Is there anything outstanding that you would like to work on?

No. Just want to thank you for your help and schedule the testing session. I have so much more energy than I used to and I'm looking forward to getting started on a bunch of things I've wanted to do for a long time.

(End of excerpt.)

When Mary returned for her testing session she announced that she was pregnant. This was particularly significant to her, as one of the reasons she chose to come for counselling when she did was that, as a result of an assault by a doctor, she had problems with attending doctors' appointments and going to hospital when necessary. She had already decided to have a home birth, but she was concerned that if something happened that required her to go to hospital she would not be able to do this. She and her husband had been delaying trying for a child until these issues were resolved. When she made this announcement, she stated, 'I'm so pleased. I'm comfortable with going for an exam and even if I have to go to hospital I know I will be fine.'

Mary's score on the PENN Inventory was 1 – obviously well below the 35 cut-off score for a diagnosis of Post-Traumatic Stress Disorder. Her score on the Impact of Event Scale was 0. At six-months follow-up, her score on the PENN Inventory was 2 and her score on the Impact of Event Scale was 0. At one-year follow-up, despite a period of intense stress in her life, her score on the PENN Inventory was 2 and her score on the Impact of Event Scale was 0. At two-years follow-up, her score on the PENN Inventory and the Impact of Event Scales remained the same as at earlier follow-up tests (2 and 0 respectively). Mary has returned for counselling on two occasions since that time – both for issues not explored during the initial trauma counselling. At that time she said, 'What continues to amaze me is that although new issues arise, the old ones – the things we worked on – don't get triggered. Resolved really does mean resolved for me.'

RESULTS FROM RENEE

Renee came in for the session following the TIR session in which she addressed the original incident that had brought her into counselling (when her husband Roger shot her), and when asked how she was doing stated 'OK'. An excerpt from the session is below.

Have you had any attention on the shooting incident we examined last time?

(Renee looks calm, relaxed.) *No. I'd rather not think about it. People keep asking about it though. I still have physical scars to remind me. They are fading now, but even a tan wouldn't disguise them. I'm not scarred by it anymore. The consequences piss me off. The incident doesn't cause me any distress now. I feel very calm now. I don't get uptight as I used to. I'm going on day to day with my life – not concerned about things like I used to. I feel OK in myself – no depressive attacks, no anxiety attacks. I haven't felt like this since before I met Roger. I spent 27 years being an object; 27 years being treated like a piece of shit on the end of Roger's shoe and then when he couldn't control me anymore he tried to kill me. He did me a favour in the end.* (Though Renee was quite calm at this point, the counsellor wanted to recheck the incident. He used TIR to guide Renee through the incident a couple of times and it was clear to both of them that there was no charge in the incident. Following this, they scheduled a session for follow-up testing.)

At the follow-up testing session, Renee said the following: 'The insight I have had is that I've been conditioned into being a soft touch. I've changed now.' When she stated this, she was smiling and sitting in a relaxed posture. The rest of the final session was spent discussing the counselling relationship.

(End of excerpt.)

Renee's score on the PENN Inventory at the post-test session was 14, well below the 35 cut-off score for a diagnosis of PTSD. Her score on the Impact of Event Scale was 21. On the PTSD symptom checklist, she no longer qualified for a diagnosis of PTSD. Six months following the end of counselling, Renee experienced a tragedy in her family life. She returned for further counselling relating to this trauma. This counselling lasted for four sessions. She told the counsellor that her life had continued to improve since the counselling and, despite the family tragedy, would continue to improve. She reported that her symptoms had not returned.

In general, TIR counselling is ended when the client's attention is no longer preoccupied with past events, regardless of whether or not all listed traumas have been addressed. A trauma, by definition, constitutes a crisis in a person's life, an abnormal experience contrasting with that person's previous experience and expectations. Trauma counselling, such as TIR, offers a way to enable a person to deal with the impact of his experience and enable him to move on. Renee provided a good example of how such a major change in her life (followed by two other traumas) meant that the manifestations of her experience required other interventions as well as considerable readjustment on her part.

Particularly for those who have not experienced substantial trauma in their lives, the impact of one (or more) can raise issues that have never occurred to them before – existential as well as practical issues. Such changes, although they can be satisfactorily addressed with brief therapy (such as TIR) to enable a person to recover from the trauma itself, may require follow-up. We have seen some trauma victims simply return to their normal functioning and carry on with their lives. For others, their trauma prompts a complete change in their thinking and life style which presents other difficulties that *may* need to be addressed. As with any other targeted intervention technique, TIR needs to be seen and incorporated into the broad view of how a person is conducting her life.

This book has primarily dealt with addressing the primary effect of trauma with a view to recovering normal functioning. The broader impact of trauma on an individual's life and how this might be addressed is covered elsewhere and is the subject of our next book.

REFERENCES

American Psychiatric Association (1987). *Diagnostic and Statistical Manual of Mental Disorders – III Revised*. American Psychiatric Association: Washington D.C., pp. 247–251.

American Psychiatric Association (1994). *Diagnostic and Statistical Manual of Mental Disorders – IV*, American Psychiatric Association: Washington, D.C., pp. 424–432.

Baker, N. & McBride, B. (1991, August). Clinical applications of EMDR in a law enforcement environment: Observations of the psychological service unit of the L.A. County Sheriff's Department. Paper presented at the Police Psychology Mini-Convention at the American Psychological Association Annual Convention, California.

Bartlett, F. (1932). *Remembering*. Cambridge University Press: Cambridge.

Bisbey, L. (1995). No longer a victim: A treatment outcome study of crime victims who have PTSD. Doctoral dissertation published by Dissertation Abstracts International.

Bisbey, L. (1996a). Six-month, one-year and two-year follow-up from dissertation research. (Unpublished raw data.)

Bisbey, L. and Bisbey, S. (1995). Workshop handout: SIR model. (Please contact the authors for a copy of this document.)

Bisbey, S. (1990). Expanded unblocking. *Journal of Metapsychology*, **III**, 7–8.

Bisbey, S. (1996b). Anecdotal follow up data on 10 TIR cases from 5 and 8 years ago. (Unpublished raw data.)

Black, J. & Bruce, B. (1989). Behaviour therapy: A clinical update. *Hospital and Community Psychiatry*, **40**, 1152–1158.

Boudewyns, P. & Shipley, R. (1983). *Flooding and Implosive Therapy: Direct Therapeutic Exposure in Clinical Practice*. Plenum Press: New York.

Brett, E. & Ostroff, R. (1985). Imagery and PTSD: an overview. *American Journal of Psychiatry*, **142**, 417–424.

Broadbent, D. (1954). The role of auditory localization in attention and memory span. *Journal of Experimental Psychology*, **47**, 191–196.

Carlson, J., Chemtob, C., Rusnak, K., Hedlund, N., Muraoka, M. (in press). Eye movement desensitization and reprocessing as an exposure intervention in combat-related PTSD. *Journal of Vietnam Veterans Institute*.

Coleman, J., Butcher, N. & Carson, R. (1980). *Abnormal Psychology and Modern Life*. Scott, Foresman & Company: Illinois, pp. 105, 107–115.

Coughlin, W. (1995). Use of TIR in the treatment of panic attacks and agoraphobia. Doctoral dissertation published by Dissertation Abstracts International.

Ellis, A. (1958). Rational psychotherapy. *Journal of General Psychology*, **59**, 35–49.

Ellis, A. (1986). Rational Emotive Therapy. In Kutash and Wolf (eds), *Psychotherapist's Casebook*, Jossey Bass Publishers: California, pp. 277–287.

Figley, C. (in press). *Eliminating Posttraumatic Stress Disorder: The Active Ingredient Symposium Series*.

Figley, C. (ed.) (1985). *Trauma and Its Wake: The Study and Treatment of Post-Traumatic Stress Disorder*, Vol 1. Brunner/Mazel: New York.

Figley, C. & Carbonnell, J. (1995, May). Memory based treatments of traumatic stress: A systematic clinical demonstration program of research. Paper presented at the Fourth European Conference on Traumatic Stress, France.

Foa, E., Rothbaum, B., Riggs, D. & Murdock, T. (1991). Treatment of PTSD in rape victims: A comparison between cognitive behavioral procedures and counselling. *Journal of Consulting and Clinical Psychology*, **59**, 715–723.

French, G. & Gerbode, F. (1990). Handout for the seminars: *Critical Issues in Trauma Resolution*. IRM Press: California.

French, G. & Gerbode, F. (1995). *The Traumatic Incident Reduction Workshop*, 3rd edn. IRM Press: California.

Freud, S. (1955). *Psychoanalysis and War Neurosis*, Standard edn., Vol. 17. Hogarth Press: London.

Garfield, S. & Bergin, A. (eds) (1986). *Handbook of Psychotherapy and Behavior Change*, 3rd edn. John Wiley & Sons: New York.

Geiselman, R.E., Fisher, R.P., MacKinnon, D.P. & Holland, H.L. (1985). Eyewitness memory enhancement in the police interview. *Journal of Applied Psychology*, **70**, 401–412.

Gerbode, F. (1989). *Beyond Psychology: An Introduction to Metapsychology*. IRM Press: California.

Gerbode, F. (1990). *The Traumatic Incident Reduction Course*, 2nd edn. IRM Press: California.

Gerbode, F. (1993). *The Traumatic Incident Reduction Course*, 3rd edn. IRM Press: California.

Gerbode, F., French, G. & Bisbey, L. (1993, June). Restoration of stability following trauma. Paper presented at the Third European Conference on Traumatic Stress, Norway.

Gerbode, F., French, G. & Van Aggelen, P. (1990, November). Pilot study of using Traumatic Incident Reduction to treat PTSD in Vietnam veterans. Paper presented at the annual conference of the International Society for Traumatic Stress Studies, New Orleans, LA.

Grinker, R. & Spiegel, J. (1945). *Men Under Stress*. McGraw-Hill: New York.

Hammarberg, M. (1990). PENN inventory for PTSD: Psychometric properties. *Psychological Assessment*, **4**, 67–76.

Horowitz, M. (1974). Stress response syndromes: Character style and dynamic psychotherapy. *Archives of General Psychiatry*, 31, 768–781.

Horowitz, M., Wilner, N. & Alvarez, W. (1979). Impact of Event Scale: A measure of subjective stress. *Psychosomatic Medicine*, **41**, 209–218.

Keane, T., Fairbank, J., Caddell, J. & Zimering, R. (1989). Implosive (flooding) therapy reduces symptoms of PTSD in Vietnam combat veterans. *Behavior Therapy*, **20**, 245–260.

Lazarus, R. (1966). *Psychological Stress and the Coping Process*. McGraw-Hill: New York, pp. 405–410.

Lomranz, J., Shmotikin, D., Zechovoy, Z. & Rosenberg, E. (1986). Time orientation in Nazi concentration camp survivors: 40 years after. *American Journal of Orthopsychiatry*, **56**, 121–135.

Lyons, J. & Keane, T. (1989). Implosive therapy for post-traumatic stress disorder. *Journal of Traumatic Stress*, **2**, 137–152.

McCaffrey, R. & Fairbank, J. (1985). Behavioral assessment and treatment of accident-related posttraumatic stress disorder: Two case studies. *Behavior Therapy*, **16**, 406–416.

McClelland, J. & Rumelhart, D. (1986). A distributed model of human learning memory. In J. McClelland, D. Rumelhart and the PDP Research Group (eds), *Parallel Distributed Processing: Explorations in the Microstructure of Cognition*, Vol. 2, *Psychological and Biological Models*. MIT Press/Bradford Books: Massachusetts.

Modlin, H. (1986). Posttraumatic Stress Disorder: No longer just for war veterans. *Postgraduate Medicine*, **79**, 26–44.

Neisser, U. (1967). *Cognitive Psychology*. Appleton-Century-Crofts: New York.

Reber, Arthur S. (1985). *Dictionary of Psychology*. Penguin Books: Harmondsworth, p. 627.

Richards, D. & Rose, J. (1991). Exposure therapy for post-traumatic stress disorder: 4 case studies. *British Journal of Psychiatry*, **160**, 161–165.

Rothbaum, B. & Foa, E. (1992). Exposure therapy for rape victims with post-traumatic stress disorder. *The Behavior Therapist*, **15**, 219–222.

Scott, M. & Stradling, S. (1992). *Counselling for Post-Traumatic Stress Disorder*. Sage Publications: London.

Selye, H. (1976). *The Stress of Life*, 2nd edn. McGraw-Hill: New York.

Treisman, A. (1960). Contextual cues in selective listening. *Quarterly Journal of Experimental Psychology*, **12**, 242–248.

Whitten, W.B. & Leonard, J.M. (1981). Directed search through autobiographical memory. *Memory and Cognition*, **9**, 566–579.

Williams, T. (1986). Psychological debriefing. (Unpublished workshop material.)

Wilson, J., Harel, Z. & Kahana, B. (eds) (1988). *Human Adaptation to Extreme Stress: From the Holocaust to Vietnam*. Plenum Press: New York.

Appendix 1

COUNSELLING ASSESSMENT FORM

This interview form is done as the first step in developing a client's counselling programme. Before the interview begins, the client should be informed that the purpose of this interview is to gather data to help the counsellor and supervisor in planning a programme that will address the right areas of the client's life. The client should also be informed that items will not be explored and resolved during this interview.

The client must be assured that all information gathered is strictly confidential and will be shared only with the supervisor for the purposes of supervision and treatment planning. (If information is going to be used in order to help in training others, the client's permission must be obtained first.)

The counsellor must remember to note the client's expression of emotion, body posture, body tone, and tone of voice as he does this interview and to make a note of emotional reactions during the interview. If an area seems heavily charged, this should be noted.

The counsellor can ask follow-up questions where more information is needed, but remember that this an assessment session, so exploration should be limited to obtaining enough detail for treatment planning. It is expected that counsellors will alter the language they use in asking the questions in deference to the client's culture.

The counsellor should attach extra sheets to this form as required.

Client's Name: _____   Date: _____

Client's Address: _____

_____

Client's Phone: _____   Client's Age: _____

Counsellor's Name: _____

1. Are you currently upset or worried about anything or anyone? (Explore and clear client's attention before continuing the form.)
2. Do you feel threatened by anything or anyone at this time?
3. Have you received previous counselling? What type and for how long?
4. (If 'Yes') What benefits did you have? Did you find any explanations or theories particularly useful?
5. Is there anything you hoped or expected to achieve in counselling and did not?
6. Have you had any other type of therapy or alternative treatment? (Get details.)
7. Are you currently involved in any other type of therapy or alternative treatment? (Get details.)
8. Is your mother living? (If 'No', get date and circumstances of death.)
9. What is/was your relationship with your mother?
10. Is your father living? (If 'No', get date and circumstances of death.)
11. What is/was your relationship with your father?
12. Have you any brothers living? (If there have been deaths, get names, dates, circumstances.) (If 'yes', get names and ages.)
13. What is/was your relationship with them?
14. Have you any sisters living? (If there have been deaths: get names, dates, circumstances.) (If 'Yes', get names and ages.)
15. What is/was your relationship with them?
16. Have your parents ever been divorced? If so, how old were you? How do you feel about it?
17. Do you have any step-family?
18. What is your relationship like with them?
19. Do you have a particularly close friend or friends? (If 'Yes', get name(s) and description of relationship(s).)
20. Were you adopted? If so, when did you find out? Do you have a relationship with your biological family? What is your relationship like with them?
21. Are you living with anyone? (If so, find out with whom.) (If sexual orientation is not clear, ask 'What is your sexual orientation?')
22. Are you married? (If 'Not') Are you in a romantic relationship? (If 'yes') Does your partner live with you?
23. Do you have any relationship difficulties with your partner?
24. Do you have any sexual problems?
25. Do you have any children?
26. If so, what are their names and how old are they?
27. What is your relationship like with your children?
28. (If the viewer is female) Other than with your children (if appropriate) have you ever been pregnant? If so, did you have the child? If

not, did you have an abortion(s)? If not, did you miscarry? (If 'Yes', get number of miscarriages and dates.)

29. Have you ever been divorced?
30. (If appropriate) How many times? For what reasons? How do you feel about it?
31. Tell me about the significant previous romantic relationships you have had.
32. Have there been any deaths that affected you?
33. What formal education have you had?
34. Is there anything you wanted to achieve and did not due to lack of or failures in education?
35. How do you feel about learning or study?
36. Are there any areas of your schooling which were rough or traumatic?
37. How are you currently making a living?
38. Are you having any difficulties at work?
39. How do you feel about your job?
40. What main jobs have you done?
41. Is there anything you wanted to do and as yet have not managed to achieve?
42. What interests or hobbies do you have?
43. Are you currently taking any street drugs? What? For how long?
44. Have you ever taken any street drugs? What? When? For how long?
45. Do you currently drink alcohol? What? How much?
46. Have you ever drunk alcohol? What? When? For how long?
47. Are you taking prescribed drugs or medicines? What? How much?
48. Have you previously taken prescribed drugs or medicines? What? When? For how long?
49. Have you had any serious illnesses? What? When? Any lasting consequences?
50. Have you had any operations? What? When? Any lasting consequences?
51. Have you had any serious accidents? What? When? Any lasting consequences?
52. Do you have any current illness? What?
53. Do you have any current medical treatment in progress?
54. Do you have any recurring physical ailment? What (such as headaches, irritable bowel, hayfever, PMT)?
55. Do you receive any disability payment or pension?
56. Have you had any unusual perceptual experiences (such as *déjà vu*, out of body experience, visions, hearing voices)?
57. Do you have any difficulties concerning eating or your weight?
58. Have you ever had bulimia, anorexia or any other eating disorder?
59. Do you consider yourself to be either under- or over-weight?
60. How much and how well do you sleep?

61. What is your usual diet?
62. Do you take nutritional supplements?
63. How would you estimate your current physical fitness?
64. Are there physical problems that run in your family?
65. Does your partner have any physical problems or disabilities?
66. Has there been anyone in your family who has suffered from any mental problems?
67. How do you feel about medical treatment?
68. How do you feel about doctors and hospitals?
69. Have there been any severe losses in your life (such as loss of valuable property, close friends, relationships, desired job)?
70. Is there anything that you often worry about happening to you or in your life?
71. Is there anything you do that you feel is not normal, sensible or logical?
72. Are you aware of any compulsions, things you feel you have to do?
73. Are there any activities, places or people you tend to avoid?
74. Do you have any fears or phobias?
75. Is there anything happening in your life that you feel unable to control?
76. Have you ever been in trouble with the police?
77. Have you any history of violent behaviour?
78. Have you been the victim of any criminal activity (such as assault/ mugging, burglary, rape, domestic violence, sexual abuse, violent life-threatening attack)? (If 'Yes', get date and details of each.)
79. Are you currently involved in any legal action (such as compensation hearings, personal injury case, divorce case or criminal proceedings)?
80. If you are involved in legal action: Is your solicitor aware that you are seeking treatment at this time? (If possible, get name and details of solicitor.)
81. Have you witnessed any severe traumatic incidents, such as war time experiences, violent crime, accidents or deaths?
82. Have you ever considered or attempted suicide? (Get details. If the client is currently feeling suicidal, find out if he/she has a plan and get the details of it.)
83. Is anyone actively objecting to you getting counselling?
84. Has anyone insisted you get counselling?
85. Does anyone not like you the way you are?
86. Is there anything about yourself that people seem to object to or find irritating?
87. Has anyone ever tried to make you change or be different?
88. What is your religious background?
89. What are your current religious beliefs?

90. Have you anything specific you hope to get resolved with counselling?
91. Is there anything we talked about in this interview that your attention is still on?
92. What is the name of your GP? What is your GP's address? What is your GP's telephone number? Is your GP aware that you are seeking counselling?

Note for counsellors: Please note the client's indicators at the end of the interview and any other observations you feel will help the supervisor in treatment planning.

Appendix 2

EXPANDED LIST OF UNBLOCKING CONCEPTS

As with the list included in Chapter 6, these concepts are to be incorporated into questions. For example, 'Regarding your relationship with your mother, have you felt powerless?' Remember that often a client will experience resolution on the issue before working through the entire list of concepts. Once an end point has been reached, the counsellor should end the Unblocking, whether he and the client have explored one concept, twenty concepts or all of the concepts on the list.

0. Effect (on client)	21. Blamed	41. Regretted
1. Suppressed	22. Compromise	42. Unrecognized
2. Powerless	23. Desired	43. Committed to
3. Distanced from	24. Concluded	44. Inhibited
4. Worried about	25. Restraint	45. Obligation
5. Wary of	26. Missing information	46. Argued
6. Misunderstood	27. Unadmitted	47. Wanted to prove
7. Disregarded	responsibility	48. Effort to be right
8. Judgement	28. Unable to control	49. Misconceived
9. Concealed	29. Advantageous	50. Misleading
10. Denial	30. Not acted upon	51. Agreed with
11. Disagreed with	31. Revealed	52. Ambiguous
12. Proposed	32. Decided	53. Unexamined
13. Incomprehensible	33. Should be changed	54. Undecided
14. Failure	34. Overlooked	55. Misjudged
15. Unacknowledged	35. Achieved	56. Unbelievable
16. Negated	36. Criticized	57. Fixed idea
17. Felt strongly about	37. Disappointing	58. Inappropriate
18. Mistake	38. Betrayal	59. Reached
19. Dilemma	39. Unexpected	60. Solved
20. Forced on you	40. Expected	

Appendix 3

REVISED SHOCK, IMPACT, RESOLUTION MODEL

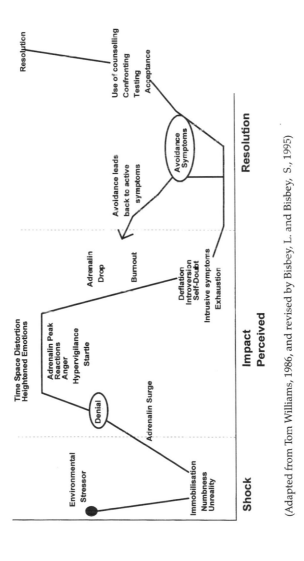

(Adapted from Tom Williams, 1986, and revised by Bisbey, L. and Bisbey, S., 1995)

INDEX

Index compiled by Mary Kirkness

Related titles of interest...

Remembering Trauma
A Psychotherapist's Guide to Memory and Illusion
Phil Mollon
This balanced review of the debate on recovered memory relates the issues to a range of psychological therapies and demonstrates the issues in practice.
0-471-97613-X   225pp   1998   Hardback
0-471-98214-8   225pp   1998   Paperback

Rebuilding Shattered Lives
The Rationale and Responsible Treatment of Post-Traumatic and Dissociative Disorders
James A. Chu
"A major contribution to the clinical trauma literature, by one of the field's most experienced clinicians."
Christine Courtois, Director of the Center for Post-Traumatic Disorders
0-471-24732-4   256pp   1998   Hardback

Treating Post-Traumatic Stress Disorder
Donald Meichenbaum
"This book will be new for years to come... it's an extraordinary volume, a crowning contribution to trauma science."
Journal of Trauma Studies
0-471-97241-X   600pp   1997   Paperback

Understanding Post-Traumatic Stress
A Psychosocial Perspective on PTSD and Treatment
Stephen Joseph, Ruth M. Williams and William Yule
Shows that post-traumatic stress reactions are not caused by the traumatic event alone, but that psychosocial factors play a vital part for individual outcomes.
0-471-96800-5   200pp   1997   Hardback
0-471-96801-3   200pp   1997   Paperback